A Patient-Expert Walks You Through Everything You Need to Learn and Do®

CHRISTOPHER LUKAS is an Emmy-winning television producer, director, and writer who specializes in films about end-of-life decision making. The author of three other books, Lukas lives in upstate New York.

THE COMPLETE FIRST YEAR® SERIES

THE FIRST YEAR®

Prostate Cancer

An Essential Guide for the Newly Diagnosed

Christopher Lukas

Foreword by Herbert Lepor, MD

MARLOWE & COMPANY ■ NEW YORK

The First Year®—Prostate Cancer:
　　　An Essential Guide for the Newly Diagnosed

Published by
Marlowe & Company
An Imprint of Avalon Publishing Group Incorporated
245 West 17th Street, 11th floor
New York, NY 10011

AVALON

The First Year® and A Patient-Expert Walks You
Through Everything You Need to Learn and Do®
are trademarks of the Avalon Publishing Group.

Library of Congress Cataloging-in-Publication Data

Lukas, Christopher.
　The first year-prostate cancer : an essential guide for the newly diagnosed /
Christopher Lukas ; foreword by Herbert Lepor.
　　p. cm.—(The first year series)
　Includes bibliographical references and index.
　ISBN 1-56924-352-2 (pbk.)
　1. Prostate-Cancer-Popular works. I. Title. II. Series.
　RC280.P7L85 2005
　616.99'463-dc22

　　　　　　　　　　　　　　　　　　　　　　　　　　2005025737
ISBN-13: 978-1-56924-352-7

9 8 7 6 5 4 3 2 1

Designed by Pauline Neuwirth,
Neuwirth and Associates, Inc.

Printed in the United States of America

PROSTATE CANCER IS THE MOST COMMONLY DIAGNOSED NONSKIN CANCER IN THE UNITED STATES. ONE IN SIX AMERICAN MEN WILL DEVELOP PROSTATE CANCER IN THE COURSE OF HIS LIFETIME. A LITTLE-KNOWN FACT IS THAT A MAN IS 33 PERCENT MORE LIKELY TO DEVELOP PROSTATE CANCER THAN AN AMERICAN WOMAN IS TO GET BREAST CANCER.

—*The Prostate Cancer Foundation*

Contents

Foreword

by Herbert Lepor, MD

THE MANAGEMENT of prostate cancer is a very controversial topic today. The list of controversies includes, but is in
no way limited to:

- ❍ Should men undergo prostate cancer screening?
- ❍ What is the serum PSA level that should trigger a
  prostate biopsy?
- ❍ How should the prostate biopsy be performed?
- ❍ Does aggressive treatment of early prostate cancer
  improve survival?
- ❍ What is the optimal treatment of early prostate cancer?
- ❍ Is there any advantage of laparoscopic radical prostat-
  ectomy?
- ❍ When should hormonal therapy be initiated for advanced
  prostate cancers?
- ❍ Should hormonal therapy be administrated chronically
  or intermittently?
- ❍ Is there a benefit to total androgen suppression?

Why do we appear to know so little about a disease that represents the second most common cancer that kills American men? Has medical science simply been complacent about this disease? The answer is absolutely not! Scientific medical literature is abundant with studies addressing the management of prostate cancer and the above-mentioned controversies. A recent Pub Med literature search I did on the topic of prostate cancer identified over 35,000 peer-reviewed articles published since the mid-1980s. But while the extensive literature provides important insights, it does not resolve the debate surrounding this condition. The chief reason for this being that studies designed to find definitive answers for how to best manage prostate cancer are difficult to conduct—they're extremely costly, require large numbers of patients who must be followed for long periods of time, and must be very closely monitored to ensure that the participants adhere to the study guidelines.

As men at risk of dying from prostate cancer and as physicians who must make decisions related to screening and managing the disease, we do not have the luxury of burying our heads in the sand awaiting the results of definitive studies. We are compelled to make decisions despite the limitations of the medical evidence. Doctors must keep up-to-date with the scientific literature, albeit imperfect, and weigh the risks and benefits surrounding the different options. Doctors must also guide the decision process for their patients, recognizing the controversies and explaining their recommendations.

Despite the questions surrounding prostate cancer (PSA) screening, an overwhelming majority of men are being screened for prostate cancer routinely or proactively. Most men will undergo a biopsy if recommended by their urologist for an elevated PSA level or abnormal prostate examination. Men and their partners begin to get actively involved in decision-making once confronted with the diagnosis of cancer, and until now there has been no single reliable resource to navigate the issues surrounding the treatment of prostate cancer. In *The First Year—Prostate Cancer,* Christopher Lukas offers you just that, by providing vital information gathered from a variety of sources, including healthcare professionals, others who have undergone treatment, and books by health care professionals and lay people as well as insights based on his own battle with prostate cancer.

Christopher's knowledge and insight will help guide you through all the important decisions you will have to make regarding the treatment and management of your condition. For instance, he encourages you—and I strongly agree—to pursue consultations from a variety of physicians specializing in different disciplines depending upon the stage of the disease. My practice in urology is limited exclusively to the surgical treatment of prostate cancer, and while I've learned a tremendous amount from the thousands of patients and their partners whom I have guided regarding optimal treatment and postoperative issues following radical prostatectomy, I've also learned that it's impossible to be unbiased. I too encourage patients to seek consultations from other experts. Men should challenge their doctors to discuss the controversies surrounding their treatment recommendations and provide a compelling reason to follow them. For those men evaluating the many different treatment options for localized diseases, they should challenge their doctors to provide and validate their personal outcomes as it relates to complications and quality of life outcomes.

Christopher advises you to seek out guidance from friends or acquaintances who have undergone treatment—the way in which they navigated their decision process can give you perspective on your own choices. Friends can also provide valuable information about the quality of care they received from their physician and the institution where they were treated.

Support groups is another important topic covered in this book and a good way to hear about personal experiences and gain insight from others who walked the path before you. Keep in mind that men who have an uncomplicated course and have been cured of their disease generally do not attend support groups. Therefore the experiences you hear about in a support group may not be representative of the universe of men having undergone treatment.

The First Year—Prostate Cancer is an invaluable resource because it discusses many of the questions surrounding prostate cancer management, provides access to other sources of information, and addresses many of the issues on a very personal level. Lukas appropriately emphasizes that this disease affects not only the patient, but their loved ones as well, and discusses how partners can play an important role in the decision and healing process. These issues are often over looked by health care professionals.

The bottom line is there is no single right answer for how to proceed with treating this disease. The best thing you can do for yourself is become educated and involved in the management of your prostate cancer. Do your best to weigh the quality of the information you gather. As Christopher points out, the good news is you will likely beat the disease. Good luck!

HERBERT LEPOR, MD, professor and Martin Spatz Chairman of Urology at the New York University School of Medicine, is an internationally recognized authority in the treatment of prostate cancer. He has authored over 250 articles and book chapters and 10 textbooks related to the prostate.

Introduction

I was in a panic. I didn't hear anything the doctor said after, "The biopsy came back positive—you do have prostate cancer."

I have cancer. For God's sake—C-A-N-C-E-R.

THIS IS the kind of statement that you hear from men who have just been diagnosed with prostate cancer. Their anxiety level is usually so high that one doctor even said to his patient, "You're going to forget everything I'm going to tell you in the next half hour. All you'll remember is that I told you that you have cancer. Don't be surprised. It's normal." Normal it may be, but it impedes your intake of possibly vital, and at the very least useful information.

This book has been written to give you the kinds of information your doctor needs you to know—and perhaps won't even think to tell you—about a disease that, when discussed a little at a time, need not be nearly as frightening as the statements above suggest.

That gut reaction

Being frightened is indeed normal, the moment you hear such a diagnosis. Of course you don't want to be hospitalized, or to be in pain, or to have embarrassing complications you may have heard or read about. And you certainly don't want to die from your cancer.

You won't die.

Or at least the chances are good that you won't.

That's the first and most important thing that needs to be said about this disease. The common phrase in the field is, "You're probably going to die *with* prostate cancer, not *of* prostate cancer."

I hope that gives you some sense of relief.

You are not alone

Prostate cancer is not a shameful condition that happened because of some deficiency of your character or negligence toward your health. What your sex life has been till now had nothing to do with it. Prostate cancer is a disease that can strike any male, and has become much more well known since such public figures as former New York City mayor Rudolph Giuliani, former senator and 1996 Republican presidential candidate Bob Dole, General Norman Schwarzkopf, former French president, Francois Mitterand, and the late King Hussein of Jordan went public with the disease. Many other famous people have had it, actors Sidney Poitier, Robert Goulet, and Jerry Orbach, and singer, James Brown.

Not to mention millions of other men around the globe.

How does your diagnosis affect your life

There are lots of other ways to calm yourself down after receiving a diagnosis of prostate cancer. And you can do that by learning about and understanding what the disease is, about how to continue to go about your life during testing, treatment, and recovery. This book will help smooth out your world so it looks familiar again, to teach you how to live *with* and then live *past* your cancer. Day by day, then week by week and month by month, I will walk you through the many issues relating to the disease, providing you with hard data, further resources to pursue, and plenty of man-to-man moral support.

But this book is for both men and women. That may come as a surprise, given that only men have a prostate gland. Nevertheless, I've written this book for readers of either sex. The reason is threefold:

Often, men are unwilling to talk about—or read about—subjects that touch on their health. Women, on the other hand, encounter and digest such information regularly, among themselves or via women-directed media. This is a generalization, but like many clichés, it's pretty true. So, if you (a man) feel uncomfortable about reading this book, you may want to ask your wife or partner to read it and introduce the details to you as she best knows you can handle them.

Even if you (a man) have bought this book yourself and have taken the time to read it from cover to cover, it always pays to have one's partner in life read it, too. After all, whatever you're going through, she will be sharing your life with you during this time and it will help you both tremendously if she becomes knowledgeable about what you may be going through. You make other decisions with your partner; this book discusses important decisions that should be made with her, too. Or him. Gay partners are not excluded from using this book; please note that, though I may use "wife" and "she" rather than the more cumbersome "wife/partner" and "she/he" formulation when discussing relationships, I mean to imply a female *or* male partner.

Prostate cancer and its treatments may alter your sex life in ways that require adjustments in the understanding and behavior of a partner, not just yourself. And, very often, that partner can find a way to help you deal with the sensitive issues that arise with prostate cancer, in ways that you simply cannot do by yourself. So it's important to share this book with your partner, to make you both aware of possible changes (which may only be temporary issues), and help keep those communications lines open.

How I discovered I had prostate cancer

When I was sixty-six, I went to Maine for a family reunion. I began to feel pain in my testicles. Not intense pain, but it worried me nonetheless. I had had a bout of lymphoma ten years earlier—put into **remission** by radiation—but it was always possible that the disease could return. I didn't think it might show up in my reproductive system; still I decided to broach the subject anyway with one of my cousins who was a physician. He suggested I see a urologist but said he was quite sure it wasn't cancer.

The pain subsided, then returned with a vengeance. Over the next six months, as the urologist did a series of tests, it got worse and worse. I took some anti-inflammatories and some antibiotics, and I worried a lot. The urologist was not concerned. He said it was something called epididymitis, which simply meant an inflammation of the **epididymis**, a long, coiled tube that stores and matures the semen from the testes.

All this, of course, was embarrassing to talk about, not to mention the actual examinations. The pain, however, was so great that I had to get some relief. When I began looking for a pain clinic, my urologist said he thought he might do another rectal examination. During that examination he felt a small hardening of the prostate and suggested a biopsy. Ten days later, while on a film shoot (that's my profession), I got a phone call. "I'm sorry to tell you," my doctor said, "but you do have prostate cancer."

It's been four years since, now, and I'm pleased to say that the treatment I got for my cancer has put it in remission—meaning it's essentially not around anymore.

And the pain? That's gone, too. I'll talk more about that when I get deeper into the book.

How to use this book

Many people have found it helpful to know huge amounts about their medical problem. Others prefer to keep it simple, and learn only as much as they can handle at any one time. This book makes both ends of the spectrum possible. You can read it through in one sitting. Or, you can read only a chapter—or part of a chapter—at a time.

To some extent, this will depend on when in the cancer process you come to the book. If it's at the beginning, just after diagnosis, you may find it too anxiety-provoking to read too much. I do urge you however, to dip your toe into the first few chapters. They can be especially helpful for those learning about prostate cancer—or perhaps any kind of cancer—for the first time. If you've had prostate cancer for a while and already undergone some treatment, you may choose, on the other hand, to use the book as a continuing learning experience, dipping in to it to find new or additional information you wish to have.

Like many health guides, this book goes into some issues in depth, while it only touches upon other topics discussed more fully in scholarly or medical tomes. In the back of this book, I list a number of organizations, books, and Web sites that can be valuable, some of which are for lay people, others of which are for professionals.

This manual is divided into twenty-one sections. The first group, broken down day by day, relate to the first week after diagnosis.

The next group relates to the next eleven months—in other words, the "year" of the title of this book.

The chapter names should not be taken literally with regard to the calendar. They are a convenient way of dividing the book into manageable sections. The first actual seven days after diagnosis may be spent waiting for further tests. Or, conversely, you may be extremely busy with tests and treatment right away, and will wish to read ahead. Your personal time frame will depend—as I will discuss in the first chapters—on what type of prostate cancer you have, where it's located, how advanced it is, and so forth.

In addition, while the book culminates at the end of the first year, many prostate cancer patients discover that theirs is a **chronic** version of the disease, one they and their physician will continue to watch over many years. The good news about this scenario: "chronic" means it's not a **terminal** or aggressive cancer. Advances in early discovery, new treatments, and technology have transformed many cancers from being potentially deadly into being manageable chronic illnesses. The bad news: you may have to undergo continuing tests or treatments as you live with your prostate cancer over a long time.

Whichever form of prostate cancer you have, you will need to see your doctor for checkups even after it's gone. This book can't take the place of that. But, from personal experience, I can tell you that it's far more preferable to go back to your oncologist from time to time for a good report than to neglect the importance of early detection and then face an immediate crisis!

One other note about the book and its arrangement. Lots of the terms in these pages may be new to you or need clearer definition than your medical consultants have provided for you. I've **boldfaced** them and put definitions in the Glossary at the back of the book.

I am not a doctor

This book is not in any way a substitute for a physician's advice. I don't prescribe medicine or recommend treatments. I will—from time to time— tell you how I dealt with *my* cancer, as well as relate to you how others have handled having the disease. But none of their stories nor mine should in any way substitute for good, attentive, and consistent medical advice geared to exactly what kind of cancer you have, and what needs you have as a unique individual. In fact, I want to state that no one should take what I say as anything but the experience and research of one man who sought answers to his own questions. You may have quite different questions. That's why I give as many resource notes as I can—so you can check out for yourself what is fact, what is fiction, and what course of action you would best choose to follow.

Learning to take control

While you may have great results in treating your cancer within a few months of being diagnosed, the focus of this book is on one year because that is usually how long it takes for a man to deal with the ramifications of this illness.

Again, the facts and lifestyle/emotional issues I discuss here do not necessarily coincide with your timeline or experiences. But read the book through anyway, in small doses or quickly as you may prefer. Why? As I said at the beginning of this introduction, getting any scary diagnosis and certainly one of cancer, can dull the ability to take things in. And I want you to take things in. To digest them. And to take charge of your own illness. Not to avoid doctors nor to overly rely upon them, but to work *with* them. The days are gone, thank goodness, when physicians said, "There, there, leave everything to me," without anything really being discussed. No wonder cancer was often a death sentence, years ago! Something health-care professionals have learned since is that, when patients feel more in control of their own treatment and illness, they do better, both physically and emotionally.

The word "proactive" comes to mind. The idea is that you won't necessarily wait for someone to give you answers to questions you haven't posed. Rather, you will want to ask *yourself* questions, and will then seek answers. You can't necessarily assume that you're getting the best advice, or that people will take the time to be forthcoming with you. Rather, you must assume that you need to ask questions, do your own research, maybe ask some questions based on what you have researched, and basically get all the information you can to make yourself feel comfortable. It's remaining in the dark about it that makes cancer frightening.

So, even if at this point you feel timid or squeamish, remember: taking control, staying in charge, will help you feel better emotionally about your disease; and will usually lead to better medical and physical results, too.

Continuing to learn

Though I have conveniently folded all this information into "one year," you should be aware that you will probably want to keep learning about prostate cancer—your particular kind of prostate cancer—for years to come. This isn't so that you will have trouble sleeping at night, worrying the cancer may come back; it's to *avoid* staying awake at night. Taking charge of your health means keeping abreast, or perhaps even one step ahead, of the knowledge that is advancing all the time.

After a year has passed, you will be asked by your doctor to come in for periodic checkups. You may want to use those checkups as a reminder that it's time to see if anything new has come out in the media or on the Internet that can help you feel more secure about your future or more convinced that steps you have already taken were the right thing to do. To periodically update your research, as well as to take stock and congratulate yourself on how well you've come along.

The Diagnosis

"IT'S NEVER too late to panic."

This phrase has been around my home for a long time. I first heard it shortly after I got married. A check had bounced, not an unusual thing to happen in a home when the husband is unemployed, as I was when we had wed forty-five years ago. However, I was not used to things like that happening, so I had a small anxiety attack. My bride, whose family had gone through numerous ups and downs in a world beset by the Depression of the 1930s and the war in the 1940s, was not one to get upset over a mere check bouncing. "It's never too late to panic," she told me, and set about getting things straightened out at the bank.

Over the years I've been married, the phrase has come in very handy. When our daughters broke limbs or split lips, it was never too late to panic.

When I was out of a job or didn't get paid, it was never too late to panic.

When I got lymphoma and then prostate cancer, it was never too late to panic.

In other words, we got through what felt like a crisis by analyzing the situation, taking whatever steps we could to deal with it intelligently, and by supporting each other.

And that's what I suggest now.

"You've got prostate cancer"

More men are diagnosed with this kind of cancer than with any other kind, except cancer of the skin. More men die of prostate cancer than of any other kind. But—most men will not die of prostate cancer. This paradox has to do with the fact that, while one in six men will get prostate cancer, it's so slow-growing—even in cases when it isn't curable—that they'll probably die of something else.

I'm going to repeat that.

While some men will in fact die from prostate cancer, *most do not*. For the most part, prostate cancer is quite treatable. This is true even though at present—and this is important—there is a lot of disagreement among specialists as to whether treatment will actually keep you living longer than if you get no treatment.

So, statistically speaking, a diagnosis of prostate cancer is not bad news. That's the good news. It means that you have a cancer that is so slow-growing that, if you're over a certain age, you may just not have to worry about it.

This doesn't mean it isn't a serious disease. It doesn't mean you needn't do anything about your diagnosis. My point is, you don't have to panic.

And, because prostate cancer is so slow growing, you don't have to do anything immediately. So, take your time. Read this book. Talk with friends and medical experts. Don't feel you need to rush into decision making.

Dealing with your initial gut reaction

First of all, try to calm down. I know that may seem a ridiculous thing to tell anyone who has just had a major shock.

When I was told I had prostate cancer, even though I'd had another, more serious cancer ten years earlier—and learned how to deal with that—nevertheless, I burst into tears.

You probably haven't previously given much thought to having cancer. I hope you haven't had it before. And no matter how much you may have read about it or known someone who has had it, the notion that you have this disease can be a terribly frightening thing. And your gut feeling is justified. You are not being a sissy if you feel mortally threatened right now. Your adrenaline is pumping into fight-or-flight mode.

But rushing to do something about your diagnosis is the last thing that you need to do right now. It feels like an emergency situation. But it is not an emergency situation.

That's what my doctor told me, when he told me over the phone that my biopsy had come back positive. He said I didn't need to rush into anything. It wasn't an emergency. Because prostate cancer grows slowly, there would be plenty of time to think about alternative treatments; even not to do anything immediately.

That didn't matter. I still cried. I was still frightened. Such brave men as Rudolph Giuliani and General Schwarzkopf were shaken on hearing they have the disease. Why shouldn't we be alarmed?

Perhaps like you, I phoned my wife and told her that I had to get together with her and think this through right away. And I rushed home. We already knew that prostate cancer isn't catching. You can't give it to someone via sexual or any other transmission. It doesn't rub off on loved ones. That means you can safely give and receive all the hugs you want from people who mean something to you. And I sure needed those hugs that day. But also, we talked, and I made an appointment to go see my urologist the very next day.

Get the facts

I realized I needed to know more. I knew nothing about the prostate gland, forget about cancer of that gland. I was so in the dark that I wasn't even sure why only men got that kind of cancer. I had a lot of work to do, to make sense of my diagnosis. So, I began to do some research. I went on the Internet, I called neighbors who had had prostate cancer, and I phoned my old oncologist—the one who had treated me for lymphoma. I wanted to know my options.

A *wealth* of options

With this disease, there are a lot of options for treatment: watchful waiting, which means regular testing without doing anything more; surgery, radiation, hormone therapy, and seed-implant therapy . . . and that's without even getting into more experimental or alternative treatments. Almost no other medical problem offers so many opportunities—and the dilemmas—of choice. Even after having had lymphoma, as a prostate cancer patient, I learned that the words "patient autonomy" never had a clearer meaning. Something I learned right away was that, following a diagnosis of prostate cancer, what you do may not be as important as what you *don't do*. And so it was of paramount importance to learn all I could about my condition and about all the methods that could apply to it, than grasp for a quick-fix solution.

I know having so many choices can be scary, too. For men of my generation (60–80), doctors have always seemed to know more than we do. With this disease, how much you can teach yourself may be more valuable than just letting your doctor make a decision for you. So you may not only feel overwhelmed right now by your diagnosis, but by the prospect of bucking a lifetime of acting differently than you may need to do now, with regard to both facing a health issue and dealing with health-care professionals. I got through it all, as scared as I was when I first began. And so can you.

IN A SENTENCE:

You've been diagnosed with cancer, but there's no need to panic.

learning

What Is Prostate Cancer?

CANCER OF the prostate is predominantly a tumor of older men (the average age of diagnosis is seventy-two). If the malignancy is widespread, it is often responsive to treatment, and if localized it may be entirely "curable." (Later on, I'll talk about what "responsive" and "curable" mean in the context of this disease.)

From the 1970s to the year 2001, the rate of diagnosis grew sharply, although in the several years since then the rate has begun to taper off. This does not mean more men have been getting prostate cancer, just that in the last thirty-odd years it has become more easy to detect and identify, and that perhaps men are going to their doctors for examination more frequently than they used to. These are all good things: the sooner any cancer is diagnosed, the more likely the patient will recover from it or, at worst, keep it under control. And in fact, death ("mortality," as the statisticians like to call it) from prostate cancer—which showed a sharp peak in the late 1980s and early '90s, has indeed taken a downward trend toward the end of the twentieth century.

For men of all races, the chance of getting a diagnosis of prostate cancer during their lifetime is 17 percent. The chance of dying of prostate cancer is now estimated at 3 percent. These rates vary depending on what age diagnosis occurs, and one's race. Black men have a significantly greater diagnosis and death rate than do whites. To give just one set of figures:

Out of every 100,000 white men over 65, who were diagnosed in 1988, approximately 900 would die of prostate cancer. Out of every 100,000 black men over the age of 65, diagnosed in 1988, approximately 1,200 would die. (If you wish to read more about this issue, please turn to Month Eleven: Living, on page 224.)

How the cancer grows

The rate of tumor growth varies from very slow to moderately rapid. But even in the latter case, those men whose cancer has **metastasized** to sites outside their prostate gland can still live for a number of years. Because most men don't get the disease until they are in their later years, if they have a slow-growing form they may not ever feel symptoms or experience problems.

Prostate cancer begins in the prostate gland

The prostate gland is part of a man's reproductive system. The kinds of cancer that attack the gland are specific to that gland.

So let's start by looking at a normal male's reproductive and urinary system. (see figure 1).

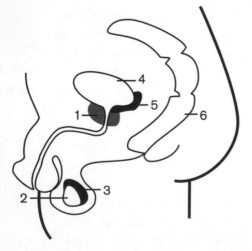

1. Prostate Gland
2. Testicles
3. Epidydimis
4. Bladder
5. Seminal Vesicle
6. Rectum

Since remarkably few men—and almost no women—are familiar with all the parts of that system, I'll begin by differentiating between parts and their roles.

The formal name for this part of the body is "genitourinary" system, because some of the organs serve two purposes: one in the evacuation of urine, the other in reproduction and sexual activity.

○ The most familiar part, of course, is the penis, which serves the dual function mentioned above.

○ Through the penis runs the **urethra**, which carries both urine and semen.

○ The bladder holds urine until it is evacuated.

○ The testes (singular, *testis;* common term, *testicles*) are protected by a scrotum. The role of the scrotum is to insulate and protect the **testicles**, which are the producers of both sperm and **testosterone**, the male sexual hormone.

○ The epididymis is a long (20-foot) coiled tube next to the testes. It is both a storage tank for the sperm as they mature, and a tube to take the sperm to the **seminal vesicles**, which are located just under the bladder.

○ The seminal vesicles comprise one of the organs that produce semen, a fluid that will contain the sperm that comes from the testes.

○ The **vas deferens** carries sperm from the epididymis to the seminal vesicles.

○ Finally, the prostate gland is a walnut-sized, ovoid structure that manufactures some of the semen. Semen from the prostate joins with the semen produced by the seminal vesicles, and together—when triggered by the sexual arousal of the man—they travel through the urethra and hence out the penis upon orgasm.

In a nutshell, so to speak, the prostate secretes semen, the fluid that carries sperm, though the sperm itself is created elsewhere (in the testicles). Lots of little pathways run to and from the prostate, the testicles, the seminal vesicles, and other apparatus in and around your rectum and urinary system.

Prostate cancer attacks the prostate gland. As you can see, the prostate is sufficiently close to other important tissues and organs for physicians to worry that cancerous cells from the gland might migrate, or spread, to other nearby areas.

The good news is that ten or fifteen years from now, if you've caught this thing early and it hasn't spread beyond your prostate gland, you'll be alive and well, and not even thinking about it. And more good news is that about three-quarters of all men with prostate cancer are diagnosed before the disease has spread.

The bad news is that just a diagnosis isn't sufficient to keep it from spreading—you've got to find out what variety of prostate cancer you have, how far it's advanced, and what treatment is appropriate for it.

But let's start with the disease itself.

What is cancer?

The easiest way to think of any kind of cancer is that some cells grow normally and are what scientists call "well-differentiated" (i.e., well-defined and shaped correctly) while, occasionally, other cells grow out of control, or change shape or size. They become what are called tumors, **malignant**. For some reason, unlike normal cells they don't accept their **DNA**'s signal to die, or they stop doing what they're supposed to do and just get bigger or multiply. They threaten to crowd out the well-differentiated (i.e., normal) cells at their original site, or spread from the original site into other areas of the body. This latter process is called metastasizing.

Cells that don't behave properly can therefore interfere with your organs and bodily functions, even with your blood or bones. So doctors need to establish as quickly as possible how far a cancer has spread, how vigorous a cancer it is, and what symptoms you have.

With prostate cancer, no one yet knows what controls the rate of growth of the malignant cells. So, while some prostate cancer is slow growing, other kinds are more aggressive. Scientists are working on ways of (a) finding out what controls the speed of growth; (b) chemical or biological agents that will slow down or stop that growth.

Symptoms

Because this cancer starts out growing very slowly, years and years can go by before the wayward cells start producing symptoms of any kind. It would be wonderful to detect the disease before symptoms begin; later in this book, we'll talk about how doctors are beginning to be able to do just that. But, for the present, most men don't discover they have prostate cancer until some symptoms appear, and many men actually experience no symptoms until the disease has spread.

Possible symptoms include:

○ A flow of urine that stops and then goes, then stops again
○ Having to get up in the night to urinate very often
○ Painful urination
○ Pain when you have an orgasm
○ Urine that contains blood
○ Persistent pain in and around the pelvic area, front or back

As prostate cancer is usually asymptomatic, meaning that there are no symptoms at all, you may have discovered your cancer through a routine test for **prostate-specific antigen (PSA)**, or simply a suspicion on the part of your physician that he/she felt a hardness or rough edge to your prostate when doing a **digital rectal examination (DRE)**.

One of the peculiar and vexing problems about prostate cancer is that even the symptoms listed above don't always point the way accurately. They could be associated with all sorts of illnesses or minor conditions, aside from cancer.

You may have had pain during urination and found out that all you had was an infection. It would go away with antibiotics, or even (if it were a bladder infection) with consumption of cranberry juice. Or, a back pain might be corrected with a visit to your friendly chiropractor or an orthopedist.

Still, if you did have any of those symptoms, they surely had you worried. They were uncomfortable. Often, they were embarrassing, too:

> Whenever I went to the bathroom, I found myself dribbling on the front of my trousers. I had to wear dark pants all the time, and send them to the cleaners every day or so. It made me feel like a little baby.—CHARLES M.

While Charles M.'s problem was an embarrassment to him, it could have been the result of lots of things besides cancer. (Some men experience this problem when taking certain antihistamines or other medications). But it was an important signal that something was wrong, and that he needed to get over his embarrassment and see a doctor. One of the things that symptoms do is alert you or your physician to the possibility that something deeper and more serious exists. Don't neglect responding to them, if only to find out that nothing much is the matter after all.

In my case, as I said in the Introduction, the pain in my testicles was what led to tests that revealed my prostate cancer, even though epididymitis is not associated with prostate cancer.

The DRE

You may have realized the importance of these symptoms when your physician suggested a DRE on one of your visits to him/her.

This slightly embarrassing procedure involves your physician putting on a latex glove and inserting a single finger into your rectum. Through the wall of your rectum he/she can feel the size and firmness of your prostate. Men over fifty are encouraged to have a DRE once a year. Younger men with a history of cancer in their family should have one earlier.

The DRE is a way of finding out whether your prostate is enlarged, one of the possible signs of cancer. I hasten to add, however, that an enlarged prostate is not necessarily malignant. You might have something called **benign prostatic hyperplasia (BPH)**, which is simply one of the unfortunate but not terribly serious results of getting older. Or you might have **prostatitis**, an infection of the organ. Corrective surgery (**transrectal urethral resection of the prostate, or TURP**) may be required for the first condition, while antibiotics might cure the other.

But they aren't cancer.

Therefore, if a DRE indicated an enlarged prostate, tests have to be done to determine if the prostate is cancerous or not. I'll get to what those tests are shortly.

By the way, if the DRE did not detect an enlargement or hard spot in your prostate, that's good news but not always definitive. Which is why other symptoms have to be noted and reported. They will lead to testing and diagnosis and a speedy analysis of which treatment will be the best defense against the disease.

IN A SENTENCE:

> *Because of its location, further testing is imperative after the diagnosis of prostate cancer.*

living

Surely the Doctor
Is Mistaken

MEN JUST diagnosed with prostate cancer may experience many feelings. One of the most normal ones is denial. This can be a healthy reaction or create problems.

Thinking the diagnosis is wrong may be a healthy response

Adolescents are especially keen to ignore their mortality—it's why they drive cars fast, leap off buildings with bungee cords attached to them, and smoke cigarettes and drink with such reckless abandon. It's why they sometimes go off to war with glee. I never thought that I was prey to that myth. I always thought I was a devout coward who knew that I could die at any moment. But when I was first diagnosed with prostate cancer, I discovered that I was playing the adolescent game. I never quite believed in death as reality. True mortality—the notion that life and death are not in our control and that we may very soon have to give up the former for the latter—comes as a great shock.

Since I don't like getting bad news, it's amazing how often I respond to bad events by saying, "It can't be!" This isn't simply a routine exclamation. It's really my mind's way of denying the reality of the accident or death or other catastrophe (or even a lesser problem—like a bad report card from your thirteen-year-old) that it doesn't want to deal with.

By denying the problem, I keep from setting into motion the body's alarm systems: panic, anger, anxiety—the "flight or fight" activities of our autonomic nervous system. This is what happened when I didn't fully "hear" my doctor's report. With one part of my mind I heard and even accepted it; with the other I denied it. And this "denial" probably works to protect you, too.

Why shouldn't we set these alarm actions into motion? They make us feel very upset; they stimulate adrenaline and other internal chemicals that shouldn't be rushing through our body without being used; and can create havoc in our lives. We want to reserve these extreme reactions for when we really need to run from a bear or when another desperate situation is actually here and needs immediate resolution. Prostate cancer does not have nor require instantaneous action.

So, denial, a kind of mental legerdemain, protects us from reacting too soon or too strongly. It's like saying, "We will take our time, thank you." In other words, "It's never too late to panic."

For most of us, most of the time, mortality is something we shut out so that we can go on with life. You can't drive a car or milk a cow or give birth to a child if your eyes are focused on your closing days. So we deny that death exists, or at least put it somewhere down the list of our consciousness priorities, bringing it up to examine in a clinical way from time to time—when we want to quit smoking or take out life insurance or run our car too close to the side of the road on a trip over the Grand Tetons. But most of us don't live with death on a daily basis; we don't fear its grip as we go to the supermarket or make love to our spouses, nor should we. We don't—as eight-year-olds do—cry out "But I don't want to die" to our mothers, only to be told "Don't worry. Don't worry. You've many many many years before you have to worry about death." Your diagnosis has now blown death's cover and brought it out into the open.

> Now, Death had come out of the closet. Now, I did have to worry about it, face-to-face, no kidding. There was a short line, and I was coming close to the ticket window. Six Barbers, No Waiting. I was going to die.—GEORGE M.

The Kübler-Ross stages

There seems to be a natural progression of emotions when terrible news occurs.

Elisabeth Kübler-Ross, who died in 2004, was the one who put this into words in her wonderful book, *On Death and Dying*.[1] There, she laid out what happens to people who are told they have a terminal illness or who hear about the death of a friend or loved one.

Kubler-Ross proposed that almost everyone goes through the same "stages," which she said are:

1. Numbness: That strange feeling of having no feelings.
2. Denial: This isn't happening to me.
3. Anger: This is happening to me!
4. Guilt: What did I do to deserve this?
5. Depression: Life is over.
6. Acceptance: I can deal with this.

As you go read this book and cope with your illness, it might be useful to keep these stages in mind, as universal reactions that are entirely natural occurrences. you should know that not all people go through all of Kübler-Ross's stages, nor necessarily in exactly the same order. For instance, you may never feel guilty as part of your response to your diagnosis. However, some men do blame themselves for getting cancer, because as intelligent beings, we want to believe there is a reason for everything that happens to us. That latter attitude is just the flip side of denial. But there is also unhealthy denial.

Unhealthy denial

There are times when we deny a problem that actually exists, and that should have attention paid to it right now. I'm reminded of the advertisement for the *Philadelphia Bulletin* newspaper many years ago. It ran in many magazines, and always included a man who was not reading the paper and who was terrified by the sudden appearance of a danger: a roof falling, a car hitting a traffic light, etc. Everyone else was reading a newspaper, with a smile on his/her face. Underneath, the caption ran: "In Philadelphia, nearly everybody reads the *Bulletin*."

Whatever the point was that the *Bulletin* admen thought they were making, what I got from that ad was that sometimes it pays to have your eyes on the street or the sky, not on your newspaper.

Which means that we should not deny the sudden existence of a lump. We should go to the doctor when we have strange symptoms. It's also unhealthy denial when we don't tell our spouse about our preliminary diagnosis of cancer because we don't want to believe it, ourselves. We might be trying to save ourselves from fear and action, when another opinion or action is what we need.

Which is why it's terribly important when you're diagnosed with prostate cancer to find out everything you can, and be open about what is happening with those close to you: Is this truly cancer? Is it early-, middle-, or late-stage cancer? Is it a virulent bunch of out-of-control cells, or a more slow-moving, better-differentiated cancer? How is this likely to affect your, and their, lives?

Men vs. women

There is a very big difference between how men may react to a diagnosis and how women may react. Men—and this is a generalization—don't like to go to doctors with "minor" symptoms. Men don't like to think that they're ill, because we equate it with being weak or not in control. It scares us to be in or anticipate being in pain; it scares us to be scared. We're more frightened of going to the doctor than are women. In fact, I've noticed that I'm a really big baby when I have even just a cold or a cut on my finger.

But my wife insists I talk with my physician when something shows up unexpectedly. For instance, when I found a lump on my neck fifteen years ago, I was perfectly willing to let it go for a while; to see if it would recede on its own. My wife sent me off to my doctor, and it turned out I had lymphoma. And by facing it, we got through it. When I got symptoms associated with my prostate, on the other hand, I was primed to go find out right away! I'd learned my lesson.

The strange thing is that this kind of cancer really does require a cautious approach. As we'll discuss later on, some physicians don't rush to treatment of any kind. They "wait and watch." So, your denial—your feeling that the diagnosis must be wrong—which comes out of a self-protective wish, may turn out to be very helpful to you in the long run. It may prevent you from rushing to treatment, rushing into expenses you don't need at this time in your life, or rushing toward anticipating a death that may in fact be well in the distance, still.

IN A SENTENCE:

Denial is a healthy response, but don't let it stand in your way of getting the facts.

How Prostate Cancer Is Diagnosed

It's time to talk about the tests used to determine the nature and extent of your prostate cancer, as well as what it all means for your future.

Major diagnostic tests

We've already talked about the DRE. What else do physicians do to find out about prostate cancer?

A lot.

The diagnostic tools of the **oncologist** (cancer specialist) are the normal tools of the scientific community: microscopes and chemical analyses. Once an enlarged prostate has been discovered by a digital rectal exam or once symptoms you report have been discussed, and if what your doctor has found is suspicious enough to warrant further testing, blood and tissue examination are the next steps.

Blood tests

These look for anomalies in your bloodstream. For instance, is there a large amount of what's called prostate-specific antigen

(PSA)? PSA is a **protein**. If your prostate is healthy, the protein pretty much remains within the gland. If it's not, more of the protein leaks out. It's not so much the amount that is a sign of prostate cancer but the increase in PSA from one measurement to the next that can ring an alarm bell. Some men have cancer despite low PSA readings. Some men with higher readings may have benign prostate hyperplasia, a noncancerous condition that affects about 6 million men a year.[2]

The PSA test is very simple to do. It requires a small sample of your blood. But—as you'll read in Day Five—it has to be interpreted with some caution. By itself, your PSA level is not a perfect indicator of the size or extent of prostate cancer.

TRUS

The **Transrectal Ultrasound test (TRUS)** employs a common medical tool—sound waves—to look at the prostate without resorting to more sophisticated X-ray techniques. It can help show the location and size of the tumor. Its usefulness as a primary diagnostic tool is low, however, because its sensitivity and clarity are not high. It's therefore used mainly to give information after cancer has already been found, or used during a biopsy to guide the physician's needle to the right spots.

Biopsies

The next most important diagnostic tool is a biopsy. To me, this is a slightly unpleasant but not terribly painful examination of your prostate. Here's how it's done: A slim tube (an **endoscope**) is inserted into the rectum while you lie conscious but with a sedative to relax you. Ultrasound equipment in the tube provides a picture of what's inside your rectum. This information is seen on a screen placed in front of the doctor (usually a urologist).

A small needle is introduced through the endoscope to pierce the skin between the rectum and the prostate. Using tiny snippers, the doctor samples as many as ten places in the prostate; he removes the tiny pieces and sends them to a pathologist for examination.

The snipping is usually described by doctors as feeling like a "pinch," but it's a little more painful than that, though not nearly as painful as many other medical procedures. I found that it was easy to put up with if I kept thinking, "He's finding out I don't have cancer."

Depending on the DRE and PSA, a doctor will take either a random sample of your prostate tissue, or check a specific area if he had felt a tumor there. Whichever selection he makes, he takes enough samples to make sure he covers the gland—though even a thorough biopsy could miss areas of malignancy.

A pathologist will examine the biopsy samples under a microscope. Normal (i.e., healthy) cells are the same size and shape, in ordered "rows." When they become cancerous, the cells and the tissue become ragged, not uniform in either size or shape.

As the pathologist looks at them, he/she will determine which are "well-differentiated" (i.e., near-normal) cells and which are not so well-differentiated. The former will get a low score (called a Gleason score), while undifferentiated and larger cells will get a higher score. Then, scores from the two areas that have the most cancerous cells will be added together. Scores for each area range from 1 to 5, so a Gleason will range from 2 to 10.

A score of 2, 3, or 4 is considered low; 5, 6, or 7 are moderate, and 8 to 10 are high. The higher the score, the more cancer is presumed to exist. And, equally important, the higher the score, the more likely it it is that the cancer may spread, because the sampling means it is already more widespread within your prostate than just a few isolated samples.

What are the most common results of these tests?

Since the introduction of a PSA test, and its accelerated use as a tool for early detection over the past decade, most men who are asymptomatic but have prostate cancer turn out to have that cancer confined within the prostate itself. By "most" is meant approximately two-thirds of those tested.

This is good news. Still, to find out exactly how big it is and whether it has spread or not, other tests may be used at this point.

Has it spread?

That brings me to the next important question for an oncologist. Has the cancer spread outside the walls of the prostate? Has it gone even further than the surrounding area; for instance, into the bones or another organ?

A number of tests may determine this but not all will be used. If a DRE has found a normal-sized prostate with a fairly low Gleason, your doctor may decide to do no additional tests. If there's a higher Gleason score, the doctor may order one or more of the following:

A *bone scan*

To detect if any of the cancer has spread to your bones, an oncologist may send you for this test. At a special facility, you will have some mildly radioactive liquid injected into your veins. This can be a little annoying because you have to get the injection, then hang around for an hour before going to lie in the scanner. The scan itself takes only a few minutes. For those who are slightly claustrophobic, you may find being in an enclosed ring discomforting. If you wish, you might want to be given a tranquilizer beforehand; discuss this with your doctor when you are scheduled for the test.

Recent research has shown that men with PSA levels of less than 10, who have no pain in their bones, probably do not have bone **metastases** "regardless of tumor stage or grade."[3] Doctors often recommend that these patients forget about having a bone scan. I had neither pain nor a high PSA, but I did receive a bone scan because I had a previous history of cancer.

CT scan

Called "CAT scan" by doctors, this is one of the most common computerized tests in the medical field these days. The CAT scan is particularly good at "slicing" areas of the body into virtual cross-sections by using a whirling set of beam projectors to take a whole set of pictures, as contrasted with a regular X-ray, which takes only one at a time. Among other things, it will be particularly useful to see if your lymph nodes have any cancerous cells.

You will be asked to come an hour early, to swallow contrast material—usually flavored with orange or mint, and to lie flat on your back as the whirling wheel circles your body.

During the test, a nurse injects an **iodized** dye into your veins. It feels very warm and may create a slightly iodinelike taste in your mouth, but unless you have allergies to iodine nothing nasty will happen. (You will be asked about such allergies prior to the procedure, and they will take precautions in case of some breathing problem, or hives, or both.)

These X-rays are developed by a computer into extremely accurate and detailed pictures of your body, segment by segment, so that any abnormality can be detected. The test, like the bone scan, can be a little upsetting to those who are claustrophobic, though most people get used to it very quickly.

In fact, the most scary thing about these tests in general are that you're having them because of cancer. Any anticipatory anxiety about the tests themselves is usually overdrawn. It is the results that count.

MRIs

This is the magnetic resonance imaging test, a procedure that uses a magnet, radio waves, and a computer to make a series of detailed pictures of areas inside the body. This procedure is also called nuclear magnetic resonance imaging (NMRI). It's most useful to show what's going on in muscles and other tissues in the body, during the bone scan.

After viewing the bone scan, the CAT scan, regular X-rays, the biopsy, and—possibly—an MRI, there are still one or two additional tests that might be ordered, but only if the doctor(s) aren't quite sure about where your cancer has spread. This would include a biopsy of your seminal vesicles, which sounds worse than it is, though all tests with needles can be frightening. Once again, there is nothing wrong with relying on a doctor-prescribed tranquilizer a half-hour before any of these tests. The National Cancer Institute (NCI) points out, as they did about bone scans, that CAT scans and MRIs—for most men—don't give much more information about your prostate cancer than ultrasound, the DRE, and the PSA. This contradicts some of what I will discuss later, all of which makes prostate cancer and its treatment a lot more complicated than it at first appears.

IN A SENTENCE:

> *There are a lot of sophisticated tests to be run to determine the size and nature of your cancer.*

The Lymphatic System

VERY FEW people know about the lymph system. Compared to the veins and arteries and muscles and bones we all hear about, it's not talked about much. But it is crucial in the workings of the immune system.

The lymphatic system is a series of very thin channels, smaller than veins, that go throughout the body, disposing of excess fluid (lymph) after vitamins and oxygen and other good things have been distributed to various organs and tissues in your body. But the system also includes tissues and organs that produce, store, and carry white blood cells that fight infections and other diseases.

The closest we get to learning about it is when a parent or pediatrician may say to a child, "Your glands are swollen," meaning funny lumps in and around your neck.

Well those "glands" are actually prominent lymph nodes that have trapped bacteria traveling through the lymphatic system. The swelling is a sign of an infection that can usually be treated with antibiotics. Lymph nodes (large mounds of lymphatic tissues) are located at crucial points along the system, filtering lymph (lymphatic fluid), taking out bacteria and other detritus, which is why they can become enlarged when infections are being fought by the lymphocytes, (a kind of white blood cell, which have a number of roles in the immune system, including the production of antibodies and other substances that fight infection and diseases.) The lymph goes back into your blood after it has done its job. The lymphatic system includes the bone marrow, spleen, thymus, lymph nodes, and lymphatic vessels. Lymphocytes go throughout the body, into all organs and vessels, looking for infection—to fight it. That's what the immune system does. They can become cancerous, and get enlarged, which is why oncologists do biopsies of organs where enlarged lymphocytes are found, as well as the bone marrow.

As you may have gathered, the lymph nodes act as part of the body's immune system in this fashion, by refusing to let bad cells or bacteria move into the bloodstream. The bad news, of course, is that cancerous cells in a person's lymph aren't benign. They are still cancer, and can grow and multiply. And they indicate that cancer has left its primary place of origin and migrated elsewhere.

living

Getting a Second Opinion

WHEN YOU actually go to your urologist or oncologist for a "first" appointment depends on how you define that dreaded hour. It can be a "first" when you merely suspect you have prostate cancer. It can be a "first" when you go for your biopsy. For me, the first appointment was when I went to see my urologist after he had spoken with his **pathology** department and learned that the biopsy (eight snippets) confirmed that I had cancer with a Gleason of six.

When my wife and I showed up for that meeting, we were both in terrible shape. Despite our gallows humor, which usually helps to keep us walking straight—a sense of humor that often horrifies our friends and colleagues—we were not in good spirits. Human vulnerability had struck us. Dr. M turned out not to be as cozy as we had hoped. In my previous visits to him—for epididymitis and subsequent related tests—his cool, professional approach had reassured me. Now, however, there was something standoffish about his attitude. Both Susan and I resented it.

This is not unusual. Doctors don't enjoy giving "bad news," even when the prognosis is good, as it was with me and with most diagnoses of prostate cancer. Doctors of a certain age have not been trained how to give unpleasant information to patients (medical schools are beginning to change that); and even urologists, who deal with the prostate all the time, don't really enjoy telling a patient that he has cancer. Who can blame them?

On the flip side of this, patients who have just been stunned with a diagnosis of cancer do not find reassuring a physician who takes very little time with them, gives them a brisk, impersonal assessment, and lists briefly a series of unfamiliar options. That's how my urologist behaved. While he started off with, "You have plenty of time to make a decision on treatment," his demeanor and subsequent language were not supportive or reassuring.

Very quickly, he told us that I could have one of several kinds of treatment, and that he would refer me to the oncologist at his hospital, if we liked. We had the feeling that he was brushing us off, though I'm sure he didn't think he was. But nowhere in the discussion—which lasted only about 15 minutes—did he suggest that "no treatment" might be a possibility, or that a second opinion might be valuable.

The idea of a second opinion has been around for a long time. But, strange to say, many, many people don't get one. I think some of this reticence has to do with people's perception that asking another physician to "second guess" their primary care doctor or his recommended specialist is an insult to the doctor's authority. People may even feel that their doctor won't treat them if he finds out that they asked for a second opinion. Another possible reason not to get another view is the wish to "get this over with." Also, people fear having to deal with the dilemma, What if the second doctor says something exactly the opposite of the first? Do they then need to get a third opinion?

If you have been told you have any kind of cancer, it is altogether appropriate for you to get a second opinion of your diagnosis. If you have prostate cancer, it's even more valuable, because it's likely that the original diagnosis came from a urologist, not an oncologist. Even if the tests have been conducted by someone who has seen dozens and dozens of cases, it still pays to get another opinion. This goes not only for the basic diagnosis, but for the treatment you might want to have, and for your prognosis.

Look at it this way: one way or the other, you're the one who is going to have to make a decision about treatment. How you choose to proceed will have an effect on your life and lifestyle; this shouldn't be about pleasing your doctor. So going with a single doctor's opinion may not be a sensible course of action.

When I got prostate cancer, even though my urologist was at Columbia Presbyterian Hospital, a major New York center for all kinds of diseases, I went back to Memorial Sloan-Kettering, where my lymphoma had been treated by an oncologist with both an MD and a PhD. There, I knew I would be dealing with a group of scientists who were doing the most cutting-edge research as well as treatment. I wanted to see what their pathologists said about the biopsy. Many cancerous or near-cancerous cells can be looked at by different pathologists, with different experience. I wanted to be sure I was in the hands of people who really knew what to look for. Later, my oncologist agreed that I had made the right choice: "Not every laboratory or pathologist has experience with every kind of cancerous cell." By the same token, your urologist or PC may not be the best expert on your particular kind of prostate cancer. For that, you need a specialist.

Even if you don't want a second opinion, your insurance company may require you to obtain one before you obtain an expensive treatment or go for a special procedure. And though that makes it sound as though they are interested only in saving money, remember that their caution may actually spare you from undergoing something your first doctor recommends but a second, perhaps more informed, doctor may deem unnecessary.

Where should you go for a second opinion?

○ You can ask the physician who made the diagnosis. This takes a little courage ("I don't want him to think I don't trust him!") but a good doctor will think nothing of it.

○ You can ask someone who has had prostate cancer where he received his diagnosis, and go there for a second opinion.

○ You can go to another physician or hospital where you've had a good experience, and ask for advice.

○ You can look for a **support group** in your neighborhood (see Month Ten for more about support groups) and see what those men have to say about trusted physicians and specialists.

○ You can visit several Web sites that deal with prostate cancer. Look for them in the reference section of this book, and use them. There's even a national 800 number from the National Cancer Institute (NCI) to help you find another doctor to discuss your diagnosis. (1–800 4 CANCER has a lot of options, and you may have to wait awhile to be connected to someone, but if you're patient you can get a cancer specialist on the line during the regular business week; after-hours you may select to be connected to lots of audiotapes on various subjects related to cancer.)

I want to tell you a little story about second opinions and why they can be valuable. Juan S. lived in a large suburban town. He discovered a lump in his neck and went to his physician, who sent him to the local hospital for a biopsy. After some difficulty in getting the sample out of the lump, the hospital's pathology department looked at it under a microscope and determined that it was not malignant: it was benign.

But Juan's wife was a nurse at that hospital, and she was not certain that their pathologists were as good as they might be. After much persuasion, she got Juan to request that the hospital send the frozen tissue to a major cancer center—for a second opinion. Weeks went by, and then one day Juan was phoned by his original doctor.

"Someone sent off a sample to another pathologist," he said, sheepishly. "And it turns out that lump *is* cancerous."

IN A SENTENCE:

A second opinion provides valuable information; don't put off or avoid getting one.

learning

Researching Doctors and Hospitals

Why not just use your primary care physician?

JUST AS you need to get a second opinion, you need to be sure that you obtain the best possible care and advice by people who have the most experience with treating prostate cancer. A general physician or internist—and even a urologist—may just not be in a position to follow through on the kinds of care your cancer requires. For example, if the doctor who diagnosed you isn't affiliated with a hospital where you can get the top-quality treatment you need, then perhaps you will want to go elsewhere, even if a physician you like and trust can't be there with you.

Besides, though you may not know this, with prostate cancer you aren't likely to be treated by your urologist or original doctor anyway. The specialty personnel surrounding the treatments you will be considering may involve radiologists, surgeons, technicians, and other doctors and nurses, none of whom would have been called in for your original diagnosis.

Plus, the field we're talking about is changing very rapidly. Clinical trials are going on all the time that are testing new—

and better—treatments. Not all doctors know about these trials or would feel comfortable recommending their results. Teaching hospitals, research facilities—these are the kinds of places where you're likely to find a cutting-edge specialist.

So, be sure to find yourself a hospital/health center and a primary oncologist who have a proven track record and with whom you're going to be comfortable.

(By the way, "comfort" isn't an easy word to define. One person's cuddly doctor is another person's "touchy-feely nerd." I've heard people say they want a doctor who is a friend; others have said they just want the best, no matter what his attitude toward his patients. Just this morning, a newspaper article by a physician asserted that it probably isn't a good idea to have a friend or longtime colleague treat you; the distinction between "best treatment" and "what my friend wants" may become confused. The doctor's professionalism may be hampered by his personal relationship with you, and consequently he may not recommend something experimental that has serious side effects. He may also feel uncomfortable discussing intimate details of your body with you or your partner, or vice versa; you need a doctor with whom you can be open and honest.)

What qualities should you look for in a specialist or hospital?

Doing research is not the easiest task. For one thing, you are probably not in the best shape emotionally to do this job right now.

For another, each person who has been treated at a particular hospital or by a particular doctor has his or her own opinion about whether the treatment was good or bad. So if you have mentioned your diagnosis to people who immediately launched into their own medical experiences, or if you have undergone other health procedures in the past, you are likely to feel a little confused about what constitutes a good doctor or hospital.

> I didn't think [Hospital X] did a good job with my son. He died.
> —Father of a cancer victim

> I really liked the treatment they gave me but they don't have a good bedside manner, I can tell you that.—Woman with breast cancer

Well, what do you want: a good bedside manner or good treatment? a friendly staff who will answer your questions without becoming impatient, or automatons who are damned good at what they do? a cozy environment, or one that appears top-of-the-line high-tech?

The answer probably is both. But is that possible? How do you go about finding the perfect blend or balance for you?

Here are some practical steps you can take:

○ Look in a manual called "America's Top Doctors," published by Castle Connolly Medical, Ltd. They've done a lot of your job for you, researching the specialists with the most experience and best training in all the major illnesses and diseases. You can see the doctor's training, what hospital he or she works at, and so on. They also list the "top hospitals," giving you information about training, the number of operations performed in each specialty, and so on. None of this guarantees you a cure, but it's a good start.

○ Call the best friend you have who has some medical experience. Ask pertinent questions: "Do you know a doctor or a hospital with a terrific reputation for prostate cancer?" "Have you found a new doctor you like?" "What do you know about my doctor, or my neighborhood hospital?"

○ Call a cancer support group in your neighborhood; ask for someone who knows the area's hospitals and physicians. Ask the same questions.

○ Get on the phone with Cancer Care, a national group whose 800 number is 813-HOPE, and that has a Web site, www.cancercare.org. Tell them your diagnosis, and seek their advice about your particular desires and needs.

○ By all means, ask someone who has had prostate cancer where he was treated. Most important, how satisfied was he with the results? You may think you don't know someone who has had prostate cancer. But, given the number of older men who have it (220,000 a year are diagnosed with the disease), it's likely that you do know someone. All you have to do is start asking, and the men will come out of the woodwork, eager to talk about their experience!

○ Finally, and perhaps as important as any of the above, find out which hospital or cancer center in your town, city, or region does this kind of work all the time. Every so often, *U.S. News* or other magazines will publish data on these matters. They will point out that experts in health care say that the best treatment—and the least amount of screwups—is usually available at the hospitals who do the most operations or other treatments for the particular disease or condition. If you need heart bypass, go where they do the most bypasses. If you have prostate cancer, go where diagnosis and treatment is done a lot. This isn't a foolproof rule, but experts say it's something to consider very strongly. If you live in a small town, you may want to use the local hospital, for the sake of being near your home and family, but do look into whether a major hospital in a nearby city has a specialist team that your own hospital lacks.

IN A SENTENCE:

Find the best doctor and the best hospital for treating prostate cancer, *no matter who usually treats you for other conditions or illnesses.*

Staging

What is staging?

LET'S ASSUME that you've gotten just the right doctor for yourself, someone who's affiliated with an institution that does this all the time. You're comfortable about the oncologist who has been assigned to you. You may even have interviewed one or two doctors to get the one you like best. But it's more likely that someone you trust has said, "Go to Hospital X. Make an appointment with Dr. Y." And you've done that.

Now begins that series of tests I talked about on Day Two. If they've been done already (by your urologist or someone else), you'll want to bring along the results or have them sent to this new doctor.

After looking at all the results—bone scan, MRI, CT scan, ultrasound, and biopsy, the pathologists at this hospital will determine at what stage you are in your cancer. This identifies where the cancer is located and how far it may have spread.

This can be a very anxiety-producing period for you. Even though I told you that two-thirds of all men diagnosed with prostate cancer are likely to have the tumors contained within or just outside the prostate gland, until **staging** has been done you won't really know. Besides, that leaves about 30 percent of men with cancer that is outside the gland, either spread to local vessels or organs (about 10 percent), or into the bones or lymph system.

I should make something clear. Not everyone gets all of the tests. How many different ones are done will depend on what was learned from the DRE, the PSA, and the biopsy. If the doctor didn't feel any lump or firm spot in your prostate, or if the Gleason score was low, it means that the cancer is almost certainly isolated within the prostate gland. If you haven't had cancer before and don't have symptoms, it's unlikely that you'd have an MRI or bone scan, but you might still have a CAT scan.

If you have a previous history of some kind of cancer, the doctor might feel it prudent to do a bone scan—to see if the cancer has spread. If you have had prostate cancer before, the likelihood is that he will order other tests to be run.

Staging the cancer

Here are the stages the medical team is looking for:

Stage I and II—Localized: Your cancer literally cannot be detected during the DRE or, if detected, is presumed to be within the gland itself. If it were not for your symptoms or your PSA, you wouldn't be getting a biopsy. But you have symptoms, or your DRE did detect the cancerous tumor.

Stage III—Regional: If your tumors have grown or spread so that they are outside the prostate itself, in neighboring muscles or canals, such as the seminal vesicles, but the cancer hasn't reached the lymph nodes or any more distant sites in the body, it's in Stage III.

State IV—Metastatic: If your cancer has reached further than that—into bones or other organs (liver, kidney, bladder, lungs) or the lymph system, then it is said to have metastasized, and is in Stage IV.

According to the National Cancer Institute—the federal government's watchdog and treatment specialists for all cancers—the latest information is that three-quarters of newly diagnosed prostate cancers are localized. About 14 percent are regional, while about 11 percent are metastatic. This is down from a figure of 20 percent that were metastatic in the early 1990s.

This is good news. It means that of the 220,000 men diagnosed in 2004, 189,200 had cancer limited entirely to their prostate gland. While those 33,000 in Stage IV don't feel that this is good news, since metastatic cancer cannot—at present—be cured (though it can be ameliorated), for the others, even in Stages II or III, these statistics are a reassuring plus.

But right now you need to know specifically about your cancer, not anyone's else.

So now is when you will visit with your doctor and get your unique test results in person, asking all the questions you need to ask, making sure that you understand exactly what you are being told. If you don't understand, ask. If you still don't understand, ask in a different way, and make sure the doctor answers in a different way.

This might be a good time to ask some of the questions that came up after your first visit but that you and your wife or partner were too shaken to bring up then.

IN A SENTENCE:

Staging brings together your test results in ways that may mean good news.

learning

What Causes Prostate Cancer?

YOU WANT to know how you contracted cancer. You may have lived a good lifestyle, eaten just the right things. You may not smoke anymore—or ever have smoked. No one in your family may have had cancer of any sort.

What causes any kind of cancer is a tricky question. "Cells start growing out of control" is the simplest answer. And why does that happen? A couple of your genes had DNA that mutated. Why? Science doesn't know yet. In the case of prostate cancer, a direct trigger has yet to be pinpointed. It's unlikely that smoking or pesticides or other known **carcinogens** are responsible; you were probably not exposed to radiation affecting this area of your body (checkups at the dentist don't count); and infectious diseases, even sexually transmitted ones, are not known to cause prostate cancer.

Here's what is known:

○ Between 1973 and 1992, the incidence of diagnosed prostate cancer increased 192 percent. This may or may not be due in part to an increase in doctors' ability to detect the illness.

○ Newly diagnosed cases began to diminish after that, but

prostate cancer now constitutes about one-third of all new cancer discovered in men.

○ If you're African American, you're more likely to get prostate cancer than if you're not, about 60 percent more. In 2001, the most diagnosed cancer in African-American men was prostate cancer (37 percent). It's not clear whether that's because of the diet of black people in America, for environmental reasons, or for genetic reasons. And, unfortunately, African Americans are more than twice as likely to die from prostate cancer than non–African Americans. Again, the reason isn't entirely clear. Obtaining early diagnosis and treatment is important, and African Americans may not have as easy access to good primary-care physicians or oncologists as do whites. At Harlem Hospital in New York City, over half of the cases of prostate cancer that are diagnosed are in an advanced stage, where the prognosis is not nearly as good as for white men.

Here's a set of graphs that demonstrate the difference between whites and African-Americans' rate of prostate cancer.

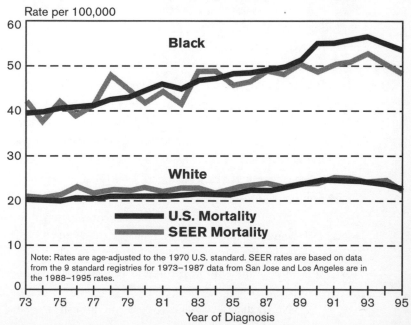

Prostate Cancer Mortality Rates 1973–1995

Other facts about the incidence of prostate cancer

○ If someone in your family had prostate cancer, you're more likely to have it. In fact, if two people in your family had prostate cancer, you're five times as likely to get it.

○ And, speaking of genetics, in 2005 a new study showed that the risk for prostate cancer is much higher if you come from a family with "a hereditary form of breast and ovarian cancer." The increased risk is estimated at about four times the normal rate, and is associated with **mutations** of the BRCA1 gene.[4]

○ If you eat a lot of animal fat (or red meat), you may also be more likely to get the disease.

○ Promiscuity *may* be a factor. A **retrospective** study from Sweden discovered that there was a correlation between men who had led a prolific sex life when they were young and the development of prostate cancer. The supposition is that once young men are exposed to the human papilloma virus (which shows up in promiscuous men and women), it engenders mutations that can eventually lead to cancer many years later.

○ Masturbation does not increase your risk for prostate cancer.

○ Efforts to find environmental factors associated with prostate cancer have proven fruitless, except for some very specific populations of people who use heavy amounts of pesticides (see Month Nine for more on this).

○ The older male population gets prostate cancer more than the younger one, but younger men (under fifty) are more likely to face a more aggressive cancer if they do get it.

○ Like other cancers, prostate cancer seems to be tied in some way to Agent Orange; at least, those who were exposed to Agent Orange are more likely to get prostate cancer than those who were not so exposed.

○ Asian men living in Asia have a low rate of prostate cancer. When they live in the U.S. for a while, that rate increases. The supposition is that environmental and nutritional factors are responsible, but no one knows for sure!

○ Testosterone is somewhat responsible for prostate cancer, but probably mainly for the cancer's ability to grow, rather than its capacity to mutate cells into a malignancy.

O It was thought that vasectomies might be responsible for some prostate cancer, but recent research suggests that is erroneous.

Note how often I used the words "some," "may," "greater," "less." The fact is, very little is known about the risk factors for prostate cancer. Which means that, at least as far as we may determine now, from much oncological research, very little could have been done to prevent your cancer.

Two of the other things most people want to know about is what role genetics plays and what can be done to lessen the spread of prostate cancer—other than major treatments, that is.

About genetics, very little is known. Your physicians will want to know if anyone in your family has had cancer, but there is little data to suggest that your father or grandfather's prostate cancer has a direct effect on yours.

And while there is some suggestion that certain vitamins—for instance, E and D, selenium, and lycopene (found in tomatoes)—may retard the growth of some prostate cancer, or even prevent cancer growth, much more work needs to be done to confirm that dietary supplements have any serious impact upon the disease.

Don't beat yourself up

Thinking, "What I could have done to prevent this cancer" may be more upsetting to you than helpful.

Suppose your father's genes *were* responsible. What difference does it make? You couldn't avoid having had him as your father. And there was no way he could have willfully imposed his genes upon you, when you were likely conceived many decades before he even knew he had cancer.

And suppose you *did* smoke: not all men who smoke get prostate cancer.

In fact, people who get this disease have little to no control over any of these risk factors, which means that you could have done everything "right" and still get cancer. Or that someone else could have all the risk factors present and not get it.

This should be reassuring to learn that you did not do anything to "give yourself" prostate cancer. It is not your fault. Moreover, it is probably no one's fault. It just happened.

IN A SENTENCE:

> *Science doesn't know enough about the risk factors for prostate cancer to know how to prevent it.*

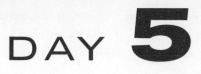

DAY **5**

You May Not Need Immediate Treatment

living

IN THIS book, I will undoubtedly repeat myself a half dozen times on one issue: whether testing or treatment makes a difference.

This rather paradoxical idea is based on a number of facts, the first of which is that PSA testing—the primary, most basic level of testing that is now recommended annually by the American Cancer Society for every man over fifty—turns up some false positives and false negatives. For instance, it has been reported that 25 percent of men with metastatic cancer had appeared to have a normal prostate upon examination, including a low PSA score.

Another controversial facet of this issue is that no completed studies show PSA/DRE screening results in lower rate of death from prostate cancer for most men.

Additionally, there is no agreement on which treatment is optimal for the localized form of the disease, nor that any particular form of treatment results in a lower death rate. Not enough has been done to compare one treatment with another over the long run. As my oncologist said to me, "The good news is they all work. The bad news is that you still have to make a choice." The word "work" simply means, the treatments probably eliminate the cancer that is now there. It doesn't mean that treatment prevents recurrence; it doesn't mean that it'll help you live longer.

Younger men excepted: treatment for men under fifty is considered beneficial, and indeed essential, since younger men are more likely to die of prostate cancer than are older men, and because prostate cancer discovered in men under fifty is usually more aggressive.

If you are over fifty, you may not need to do anything right away. Or perhaps, ever.

Watchful waiting

"Watchful waiting" is defined as refraining from any active treatment unless or until the disease begins to progress. Knowing when it progresses is a tricky matter, but six-month PSA tests, DREs, and perhaps biopsies are indicators.

This "treatment" doesn't do anything but watch your condition. It is used primarily for the two-thirds of men who have prostate cancer at Stage I or II. It is based on the assumption that your cancer is very slow growing and will not—in its present form and size—be the thing that kills you. It is also based on the assumption that it is possible to overtreat as well as undertreat you.

In the early days of treating prostate cancer, surgery was the only option, and most diagnoses were soon followed by a complete removal of the prostate gland. We now know this to be an extreme and unnecessary measure for many men experiencing only Stage I or II.

In recent years, specialists have widened the range of treatment, and very often prefer to take a wait-and-see attitude toward the cancer. It is in fact a treatment option, not a failure to treat: while no specific medicine or other procedures are being used to reduce or eliminate the malignancy, the oncologist is observing, measuring, and carefully calculating whether your particular kind of prostate cancer needs anything else done to prevent its growth or spread.

How is watchful waiting done?

This treatment option requires you to do nothing but see your doctor every six months or so for him to assess your condition. Your doctor will reassure you from time to time that this is a very slow-growing cancer and will not kill you.

He may also tell you that he doesn't really know at what stage the risk of treatment is greater than the risk of waiting. "Risk of treatment" refers to the side effects and possible dangers of surgery or radiation.

He will tell you that there is little doubt your cancer will be eliminated if the prostate is taken out, but that such an extreme measure may be premature or unnecessary, and may create undesirable complications.

The benefits of watchful waiting are numerous, but the most important are:

○ You don't need to make any decision right now about which of the more advanced procedures you want to have—all of which have some benefits, but also some drawbacks.
○ You can go about your normal life.
○ Some new treatment may come along that will allow you to avoid surgery and/or radiation.

The main drawback to watchful waiting is that your tumor may advance during this period and become a more serious form of prostate cancer.

Clearly, you and the doctor will want to discuss all the reasons that he feels waiting is a good idea. Here are the conditions under which watchful waiting is now considered a reasonable option:

○ You have a low Gleason score.
○ Your cancer has not progressed outside of the gland itself.
○ If your health isn't very good for other reasons (this is called "co-morbidity"), you may find it worthwhile to avoid treatments that may put a burden on you physically, not to mention emotionally.
○ Your PSA hasn't leapt upward in the last year.

By these criteria, a man with a Stage I cancer with a Gleason of 2 to 4 would be considered a good candidate for watchful waiting: his cancer is very slow growing; it hasn't spread; and he can probably find out—with periodic PSAs, DREs, and (if necessary) another biopsy—long before it does.

Other factors concerning this option

How old you are, whether you're in a sexual relationship, and what you do for a living may also play a role in whether you decide to watch and wait or proceed with other options.

○ The older you are, the less likely the cancer will spread before some other disease kills you. I know this sounds blunt, but if you're over seventy-five, with a low Gleason, there's a good chance you won't ever have prostate cancer serious enough to kill you. As for other age-related specifics, see below.

○ If you're active sexually, you may want to think twice about other—more aggressive—options because of the danger of impotence.

○ If you're a very active person, again with low Gleason and a Stage I cancer, you may find it beneficial to watch and wait, rather than pursue treatments that will interfere with your current lifestyle.

How does age factor in?

Prostate cancer is different from almost all the other cancers, in that it is very slow growing: So slow, that a man of thirty-five who has some cancerous cells in his prostate will live another fifteen years before the tumor doubles in size. So slow, that men in their seventies and eighties will almost certainly die of something other than prostate cancer, even if they don't get treated. So slow that watchful waiting without any additional action may last a man's lifetime.

Younger men—in their forties through sixties—may see their prostate cancer grow or spread in twenty or thirty years to the point where it becomes dangerous or even beyond treatment. But most of the men whose prostate cancer is discovered and diagnosed are in their later years, which offers more protection against death from this form of cancer.

Why is the research so vague about mortality?

We don't know enough about the rate of death from prostate cancer because no long-term studies comparing various treatments—as well as watchful waiting—have been completed.

They have been started, but because prostate cancer wasn't a major area of concern until relatively recently, and because long-term studies for prostate cancer have to be *really* long-term, lasting decades (because the cells grow so slowly), those trials are only in their middle stages.

Which means: oncologists can't tell you for sure that you'd be just as well off not getting treatment as getting treatment. They can't claim that any substance or lifestyle change will absolutely prevent the growth or spread of prostate cancer. They can't tell you that any particular treatment will change the age at which you will die, perhaps of totally unrelated causes. All they can tell you is that, if the tumor is in an early stage, it may be many years until it advances, if ever. So watchful waiting may be a sensible option for you and your oncologist to take, in the face of all those other uncertainties about the benefits of treatment.

Two things to keep in mind if you choose watchful waiting:

1. You may be able to live for many years with no additional symptoms or signs of disease. When I say "years," it could be as many as ten or fifteen years. In fact, it is very possible you will die of something quite different from prostate cancer.

2. Just because you choose watchful waiting doesn't mean you don't have to see your doctor and go through periodic additional tests. Also, you need to be able to bear the emotional brunt of knowing there is a cancer "down there" despite your doctor's reassurances that you are doing fine. In other words, if you're worried to the degree that you will avoid being tested regularly for fear of bad news, or you feel as if you are a walking time bomb rather than that the situation is under control, then watchful waiting may not be for you.

IN A SENTENCE:

> *Before you do anything, discuss with your doctor whether you even need to do anything.*

learning

The PSA Test

The doctor told Milken, then 46, that he was too young for prostate cancer to be a threat and declined to give him the PSA test. Milken insisted: "Humor me—I can afford it." The test came back with a PSA level of 24. A biopsy revealed the worst. An MRI and other scans showed that the cancer had spread to his lymph nodes, though not yet to his bones.—from a November 2004 *Fortune* magazine article on Michael Milken.

The PSA controversy

We now start down a slippery slope of controversy.

In some ways, this section of the book could be considered one of the most important. Until now, I've tried to present *facts:* those things you need to know about prostate cancer that have a high level of investigation and proof behind them. By this chapter, you've learned who is most at risk for prostate cancer, what won't prevent it, what a Gleason score can tell you, which diagnostic tests are used, and what the various treatment **modalities** are.

As you may recall, I've also noted that the PSA test is not the best diagnostic tool. But I haven't yet told you all the reasons why. Here's the bad news:

While at present there are **randomized** clinical trials in the United States and Europe to determine if there is a benefit associated with PSA screening, it is not yet known if having such screening actually reduces the rate of death from prostate cancer. And, more important, although PSA screening can lead to biopsies, and the biopsies can lead to diagnosis and treatment, it can also lead to false positives or, equally sad, treatment that isn't *necessary*. To make decisions even more difficult, treatment in and of itself may not limit mortality.

How can this be?

Scientists don't want to claim that a treatment can save lives unless they can *prove* it. And they don't want to say that a *screening* causes greater good than doing nothing unless they're sure about *that*. One's commonsense assumption is that having a screening that shows cancer—and then eliminating the cancer—*must* save lives, but the medical community does not, in fact, have such proof.

Here's what the NCI says about this crucial matter:

> The evidence is insufficient to determine whether screening for prostate cancer with prostate-specific antigen reduces mortality from prostate cancer. Screening tests are able to detect prostate cancer at an early stage, but it is not clear whether this earlier detection and consequent earlier treatment leads to any change in the natural history and outcome of the disease.

Since screening for prostate cancer may lead to diagnosis at earlier and earlier stages, and since it is not known whether such screening and treatment actually saves lives, researchers are even now studying this matter. The NCI-supported Prostate, Lung, Colorectal, and Ovarian Cancer Screening Trial (PLCO) is designed to show whether screening tests can actually *reduce* the number of deaths from these cancers. The prostate cancer screening tests currently under study in the PLCO are the PSA and DRE. The researchers will continue to screen men in its study until 2007, and then will analyze the results. The trial will directly assess the harms and potential benefits of routine screening for prostate cancer. The results of this trial may change the way men are screened for prostate cancer.

So, we are still a few years away from any answers.

How doctors view the PSA test

While my urologist, and perhaps yours, believed enough in the PSA and attendant diagnostic tools to do a biopsy, it turns out that not all urologists agree on whether to screen using PSA. The NCI reports that many different factors affect the likelihood of a recommendation for prostate cancer screening from a physician. In one study, 714 doctors responded to a request for information. Of those, 68 percent said they always recommend PSA screening. According to the NCA, "The survey results suggest that gender (male), age (medical school graduation before 1974), and mode of reimbursement (fee for service) all increase the likelihood of PSA screening among this population."

What are the cons of using the PSA for diagnosis?

As I suggested above, according to the NCI, "The possibility of identifying an excessive number of false positives in the form of benign prostatic lesions requires that the test be evaluated carefully." In other words, if the test has a documented history of interpreting nonmalignant tumors to be cancerous, possibly resulting in unnecessary treatment (not to mention unnecessary worry on the part of the patient), why screen?

We need to keep in mind that the PSA also has a **false negative** rate: there is no way of assuring a man who has a very, very low PSA value doesn't have cancer; the present PSA test may just not be sensitive enough to tell us anything. So, the test may give that man a dangerous reassurance that the coast is clear.

Finally, another factor that muddies the waters is that different laboratories may use different standards when processing PSA samples, so that one sample one year may not be properly compared with a reading in another year.

Where the medical community now stands on the PSA

While in October 2004, only a small number of oncologists and urologists were advising against use of the PSA, and others were definitely for it, by June of 2005, the picture had changed. The man who invented PSA testing twenty years ago says it's "overused" and, therefore, useless. The American Cancer Society says it's worth having every man over fifty tested with the PSA once a year. The National Cancer Institute is far from declaring anything like that.

This is a crucial, if startling, statement. It seems as if the whole basis on which thousands of men have been screened is not a good one. It seems as if thousands of men may have been *treated* for prostate cancer without good reason. Yet it is only recently that the medical profession—and the media—have realized and acknowledged this revelation. In the *New York Times* of June 20, 2005, a special *Men & Health* section stated this "discovery" in bald, unequivocal terms.

" . . . last month, Dr. Peter C. Albertsen of the University of Connecticut Health Center published a study in the *Journal of the American Medical Association* saying men with prostate cancers that do not look particularly aggressive under a microscope—the majority of men whose cancers are found with PSA tests these days—can do perfectly well with no treatment for at least 20 years."

"Most men eventually develop prostate cancer, but most of the time it grows so slowly that it never causes problems."

" 'As we repeatedly biopsy men, we are likely to find . . . subclinical prostate cancers . . . we will label more people as abnormal, telling them they have cancer and throwing them into a terrifying whirl of decision making.' " [Dr. Timothy Wilt, professor of medicine at the Minneapolis Medical Center.]

What are the negative factors? Summing up:

○ The test finds too many slow-growing cancers that don't need treatment.
○ PSA levels can rise from benign conditions.
○ PSA levels, by themselves, don't distinguish between benign and malignant conditions.
○ Hormone therapy can lower the PSA levels as reflected in the test, but don't necessarily reflect the presence or absence of cancerous cells.
○ Thus, there are both false-positive and false-negative PSA tests.
○ The PSA test causes men to worry about the presence of prostate cancer in their bodies when they may not need to worry. That can

lead those men to have unnecessary biopsies or get treatments for early-stage/slow-growing tumors when they don't need to do anything but watch and wait.

What are the counterclaims by those who advocate the test?

○ New variations on the test—new **markers**—are being developed yearly. One, called the "percentage of PSA," looks at a ratio: the relationship between what is called "free-floating" PSA to the total amount of PSA attached to proteins. By looking at a *ratio* rather than an absolute figure, oncologists believe they may have a better measure of the significance of PSA numbers.

○ New studies are looking at the relationship between a man's PSA density to the size of his prostate, hoping that this will give a more accurate reading and predictor of cancer.

○ The PSA is useful in finding aggressive prostate cancers—especially in younger men (forty to fifty-five)—that otherwise might not have been discovered early enough to treat successfully.

○ If we go back to a time when the PSA wasn't in use, we go back to a time with higher rates of prostate cancer deaths. Reports have now come out that men with a low pretreatment PSA are less likely to have a relapse within five years than men with a high pretreatment PSA.[1] For some men, this alone would make it worthwhile at least knowing their PSA. But would it help with deciding which treatment, if any, for you to get? I must leave that up to you.

But doesn't early treatment save lives?

I've said—and most oncologists agree—that all of the treatments for most men with prostate cancer are pretty much equally effective. "Effective" means that those treatments can get rid of the prostate cancer in most cases where it is now located. Even if it comes back, it'll be amenable to some more treatment. The exceptions, of course, are those men with more aggressive tumors that have escaped the prostate itself, metastasized into bone or lymph nodes. For them, treatment may slow down the growth of tumors and help with pain. But it isn't at all certain that those treatments save lives.

We cannot say definitively that any specific treatment will actually give added years of life to men with prostate cancer. So the PSA may simply result in a lifetime of worry and expense that won't change a thing.[2]

An analogous situation are the tests for Alzheimer's disease. There are some genetic markers for that frightening disease. You can, in short, be tested to see if you might be a candidate for Alzheimer's. But what if you found out that you were? There is nothing you can do about it at present. Do you want to live with the anxiety that, every time you forget where you put your coffee cup, you have the disease?

That is why some physicians say, "Don't use the PSA." One physician who appeared on a television program about prostate cancer in 1997 said that the danger from having a test like the PSA is that it can lead to the biopsy and other tests that "label" the patient as a cancer patient for the rest of his life.[3] But, the doctor said, there is no proof that that information is useful. He added, "If the patient has no symptoms, then why bother?" Why start people down the path of anxiety if we don't know that treatment will make them live longer?

But women have mammograms and those create anxiety

Yes, women have mammograms, because this screening can show that breast cancer is present. Such testing is important (though how often it is done remains controversial) because those tumors grow relatively quickly, and because long-term studies have shown that treating breast cancer does save lives.

What about quality of life, if not length of life?

Clearly, as with all controversies, there are some cases in which finding out exactly how much prostate cancer is in your body and where it is, can be important. If you're in pain, if you have symptoms, if the cancer has spread, you do need to know you have a tumor, and you will want to do something about it!

Some studies have begun to show subtlety in the range of PSA scores that can indicate size and possible aggressiveness of prostate cancer, so again part of the answer comes down to using an oncologist with access to the most up-to-the-minute information with which to interpret your score.

PSA *velocity*

Experts generally agree that when the test was first put into widespread use in the 1990s, it picked up a lot of advanced cancers that had previously been missed.

An article in *HealthDay*, an Internet newspaper, points out that, "As annual screenings have become more commonplace, PSA screening is now detecting much smaller cancers—many of them slow-growing and worthy of 'watchful waiting' rather than more radical prostate-removing surgery."[4]

Experts interviewed by *HealthDay* say that what has to happen is researchers need to become more sophisticated about the biochemistry of the PSA test, to "differentiate prostate cancers that are more likely to be aggressive and to cause problems from the slow-growing tumors that are often found."

This November 2004 article was responding to a Dutch clinical study that came down heavily in support of watchful waiting.

The study found that in some men with prostate cancer, their PSA levels don't get higher; they may even decrease. What this means isn't yet known, but the researchers suggested that relying entirely on the PSA is a mistake, and that holding off on treatment certainly is worth considering.

In the beginning, too, when the prostate-specific antigen was discovered, the PSA test was used to determine if surgery or other treatment had done its job. The idea was that the antigen wouldn't be there if the prostate itself was removed and all cancer cells had been taken out with the surgery.

Then, doctors began to discover that PSA levels in the blood could predict the presence of cancerous cells in and around the gland—more or less.

They came to see and believe that the higher the PSA score, the more likelihood that cancer was in the prostate. A high level, by the way, has come to mean 4 nanograms or greater as a trigger for a prostate biopsy.

Recently, the concept of "PSA velocity" has come into play. This means looking at the change in PSA levels across months. A large and quick increase in PSA might suggest cancer.

And they also began to see a difference in the kind of prostate cancer based on rapid PSA velocity, as possible evidence of an aggressive disease.

That's it. Get further tests if your PSA is over 4. But keep in mind that PSAs can go up to 50.

Why get tested if it's as low as 4?

Even men with low scores need to be watchful of "PSA velocity." The American Cancer Society (ACS) reports a recent study that shows that a rapid rise in PSA could be a predictor for the presence of aggressive prostate cancer. The ACS also says that some men with low PSAs have prostate cancer.

Let me repeat that age makes a difference here. Younger men stand more to gain from the PSA test than older men, because younger men have potentially far more years during which an aggressive cancer may grow and spread.

What still isn't known is whether aggressive cancer in younger men can be stopped, or at least for how long. The *Fortune* article about Milken has a long tale to tell about him.

The short version is that he did get a biopsy after his PSA was found to be highly elevated. And he did opt for treatment.

Should you be tested?

One nonpartisan expert suggests you consider the following three questions before having your PSA tested:

1. What if the PSA *were* elevated? What would you do then?
2. What if you *have* prostate cancer? What would you do?
3. What real difference would it make for you to know?

You definitely need to discuss the cons of the test with your doctor, and be sure that he is aware of them. According to the National Cancer Institutes Prostate Cancer Web site,

> At a minimum, men should be informed about the possibility that false-positive or false-negative test results can occur, that it is not known whether regular screening will reduce deaths from prostate cancer, and, among experts, the recommendation to screen is controversial.

What is known

A few things can be stated with certainty.

○ Younger men (under fifty) need to look at the PSA, as well as treatment, differently than men over seventy.
○ If the cancer is localized, and your age is advanced, you should certainly talk with your doctor about not actively pursuing PSA as a "gold standard" of diagnosis or prognosis.
○ You should keep abreast of advances in the use of the PSA, as well as new tests that refine or replace it.

On a personal note, my PSA was never above 4, though my urologist felt a small bulge in my prostate and did the biopsy that discovered my cancer with a Gleason of 6. I did have treatment (radiation), and I do get a yearly PSA. But remember, I also had lymphoma some years back, so the possibility of other cancers roaming around my body is more likely than someone who has not had them.

Let's return to Michael Milken. What would have happened if he had not had a PSA test? We can't know. But here's how he handled his aggressive cancer:

> Milken told his doctors at Cedars-Sinai Hospital that he wanted an aggressive course of treatment to clear any malignant cells from his lymph nodes and prevent their spread to the bones. That meant hormone therapy, which consists of giving patients estrogen or an "anti-androgen" drug—both of which interfere with the production of testosterone, a male hormone that prostate cancer cells require to proliferate. For months Milken took two pills three times a day, plus a monthly injection. When that was over, he underwent eight weeks of radiation therapy.[5]

Soon, he was in remission.

IN A SENTENCE:

> *Discuss with your oncologist whether a PSA test may be beneficial or needlessly worrisome for you.*

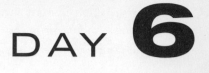

Is Surgery Appropriate?

SURGEONS LIKE to operate. Before you submit to the knife, it would be wise to know what they do and why they do it.

Surgery has come and gone as a popular way to deal with prostate cancer. From the mid-1980s up into the early '90s, about a third of prostate cancer patients were operated upon. This was six times the percentage that had surgery in 1984, and was true for men from age sixty-five to eighty-eight. But since 1993, the NCI reports the rate of surgery has been dropping.[1] I'll get to the reasons behind this later.

What is this kind of surgery called?

The operation is called a prostatectomy. Like any word that has "ectomy" at the end, that means a complete removal of the organ. This can be done in a number of ways, with incisions in a variety of places, depending on the preference of the surgeon. The procedure usually involves a hospital stay of several days.

According to the National Cancer Institute's Web site on prostate cancer,

> In a radical prostatectomy, the surgeon excises the entire prostate gland, along with both seminal vesicles, the enlarged lower sections of the vas deferens, and other surrounding tissues.

The section of urethra that runs through the prostate is cut away (and with it some of the sphincter muscle that controls the flow of urine).

No wonder that the word "radical" is used to describe this operation.

The value of surgery

The most obvious plus for patients who have a prostatectomy is that it removes the entire cancerous gland and some surrounding tissue. For the three-quarters of the men whose cancer has remained contained within the prostate (i.e., Stage I and II patients), this surgery removes the cancer.

Possible problems after surgery

It is not unusual for side effects to include partial urinary and/or bowel **incontinence**, and **impotence**. Even as surgeons' techniques have improved, and have become better at avoiding the nerves that control urinary and erectile functions, recent surveys indicate that:

○ Two-thirds of surgical patients reported problems with urinary incontinence.
○ One-third needed absorbent pads to cope with wetness.
○ Sixty percent were unable to have an erection.
○ Twenty percent needed treatment to "relieve urinary complications caused by scar tissue in the urethra."[2]

While some of these side effects reverse themselves with time, and the new techniques mean that their occurrence is less likely than in the past, these surveys are not pleasant to read.

Because it is almost impossible to determine ahead of time whether crucial nerves can be avoided, just who becomes impotent afterward is almost indeterminable. Some doctors won't even give odds on such side effects. Some who do provide a number say that there's a 90 percent chance; others suggest a much lower figure.

In addition, especially in older men—though in small numbers—such complications as infection, bleeding, and heart problems have resulted from this kind of surgery.

In younger men who still want children, there is no possibility of fathering offspring after a prostatectomy, because the prostate creates the seminal fluid, and that will no longer be manufactured after the prostate is removed, even if erectile function itself is unimpaired.

Then why is this a popular option?

The fact that surgery has remained a popular choice for up to 30 percent of prostate cancer patients is due to several factors:

○ Our propensity in this country for wanting a "quick fix."
○ Our desire to get "all the cancer" out at one time.
○ Historically, the medical profession has preferred to "overtreat" rather than undertreat.
○ The fact that patients often first hear of treatment options from their urologist—many of whom are also surgeons—and go with his opinion.
○ The anxiety associated with watchful waiting is eliminated.

What if the cancer is not localized?

Stage III patients, you will recall, have a tumor that has extended beyond the prostate itself, perhaps having invaded the seminal vesicles. In Stage IV cancer, the malignancy has spread to the lymph system or bones, or perhaps to such organs as the bladder, liver, or lungs.

In Stage IV cases, surgery alone will not stop the spread of the cancer, will not eliminate cancer in the bones or lymph systems, and will not stop further metastasis or pain associated with bone cancer.

In Stage III cases, while surgery can eliminate the basic seat of the cancer, surgeons will also need to take out any other possibly affected tissues and vessels, and continue treatment with radiation.

However, this being said, it is most likely that many men with Stage III or IV prostate cancer will opt for surgery, since the side effects associated with the operation are going to be considered less problematic than possible spread of the cancer.

What about stage I and II cancer?

When it comes to localized tumors, whether to go with surgery is more difficult to assess.

A major reason to elect a prostatectomy seems to be: "If I can get it all out, why *not* go with surgery? Why not be sure?"

There's nothing wrong with being sure, but there are a lot of things to be sure about:

○ Are you and your doctor sure that your cancer is spreading fast enough to cause real concern about your health?

○ Are you sure that other treatments might not slow it down or even stop it—treatments that might be less extreme?

○ Are you sure that you want to risk impotence and/or incontinence, infertility, or other complications of surgery?

○ Are you sure that you have the best opinions and have thought through the best options?

○ Are you sure that your **quality of life** will be improved by the surgery?

○ Are you sure that prostatectomy will extend your life by x number of years?

Since some studies have found that for the next ten or fifteen years of a man's life, watchful waiting is not substantially different in terms of life expectancy than is surgery, these questions are worth considering at this time.

I will get into this in greater depth later. Nothing in this arena is as simple as it sounds, but the fact that men are choosing radical prostatectomy a little less these days may reflect some of the new information that is circulating about these matters.

Quality of Life

IN THE PAST ten years, the notion of quality of life has taken a strong hold on the field of medicine. It is tied up with the notion of **palliative** care, which aims to relieve suffering, to strengthen relations between patients and their loved ones, to focus on emotional and spiritual issues, as well as to eliminate pain from painful illnesses.

Among other things, quality of life means that a patient defines how he wants to live when he is hit with a serious illness. You decide how you want to deal with your pain or other symptoms, and how you want to be treated in and out of the hospital.

If surgery, for instance, will interrupt and reduce your enjoyment of life, and won't increase your life expectancy, it's up to you to decide whether it's worth doing. If, on the other hand, the attendant anxiety at not "getting it all out" would make your life less enjoyable or bearable, you have the right and the responsibility to make that decision.

Each person's quality of life, in other words, must be self-defined. Some thoughts to consider:

○ How free will your choice leave you to enjoy your preferred lifestyle?
○ What impact might your choice have upon your partner or other family members?
○ How will your choice affect your job, if you are still working?
○ How important is it to you to get your illness under control, once and for all?
○ Conversely, can you bear the thought of allowing a tumor to remain within your body while you watch and wait, or pursue other forms of treatment?
○ Is the idea of being in the hospital or having surgery—for anything—frightening to you?
○ Is being incapacitated even briefly by anesthesia or painkillers disturbing to you?
○ On the other hand, do you prefer as much sedation as possible for physical pain?

○ Could you deal emotionally with such side effects as incontinence or impotence following a prostatectomy?

○ Do you desire to father a child?

One man may say, "I've got too much stuff to do, too much life to live. Operate and let me move on." Another may have as vigorous a life, but may wish to avoid going into a hospital, being in pain or sedated during surgery or recuperation, or having to deal with the possible long-term side effects of surgery. Another form of treatment may better suit the latter's emotional or familial needs.

Only each individual can tell if surgery is the right decision for him.

IN A SENTENCE:

For many years, surgery has been the main option for prostate cancer, but you do have other, less-invasive options.

learning

FAQs about Prostate Cancer

IT MAY be helpful to have some of the most prominent questions about your cancer here in one section.

Who gets prostate cancer?

Only men can get prostate cancer, because only men have a prostate gland.

The following can be said about the disease in detail:[3]

○ It afflicts one in six men in their lifetime. Men are diagnosed with prostate cancer 30 percent more often than women are diagnosed with breast cancer.
○ It is present in more than 9 million men.
○ It kills one man every 13 minutes.
○ It is second only to lung cancer in annual cancer deaths of U.S. men.
○ It has a higher risk for black men—they have incidence and mortality rates as much as 50 percent higher than other racial or ethnic groups.

How do I know I have prostate cancer?

Unfortunately, you probably don't unless you've had some symptoms that sent you to your urologist. But these symptoms could come from other problems, so unless your doctor does some tests on you, you may not suspect or know for sure that you have this disease.

Once the test results are in, your doctor will have enough information to make a diagnosis.

How did I get prostate cancer?

No one knows why prostate cancer occurs. We do know that it is very, very common. Fifty percent of men over seventy get it, and 75 percent of men over eighty have it. In fact, it's the second most common cancer for men to get (skin cancer being first.)

On the other hand, we do know what *doesn't* cause it. We know that sexual practices don't cause it. We know that other lifestyle practices don't cause it—even drinking and smoking and illicit drugs, which are responsible for many human medical problems.

How about nutrition?

There are lots of people who will tell you that what you eat does affect whether you will get prostate cancer. But the National Cancer Institute (NCI) doesn't seem to believe that. Sure, it's healthier if you eat balanced meals, if you stay away from animal fats (under 20 percent), and consume all those greens and fruits that are recommended for all of us these days. But what you eat or used to eat probably did not cause you to contract this disease.

But there are books out there . . .

Yes, there are books in the marketplace that tell you that nutrition is key to getting or treating prostate cancer. I can only repeat that most scientists don't think that's true.

Can my partner get prostate cancer from me?

The answer is categorically no. No known transmission of any form of cancer occurs from person to person, no matter how intimate the contact. It is true that you may experience pain from having anal intercourse if you have prostate cancer or are being treated for prostate cancer, but that would be true of prostatitis or benign prostatic hyperplasia, too. The cancer itself is not contagious.

Will I die from my prostate cancer?

The likelihood is greater that you will die from something else than from this disease. That's especially true if the disease is in an early stage, if it's got a low Gleason, if you are not under forty, and if your health is generally good. Yes, some men do die from prostate cancer, about 35,000 a year. But that number is beginning to drop, and considering that millions of men have the disease, that's a very low number. It is very important to your emotional well-being to break free of the mind-set that cancer inevitably results in death.

What kinds of treatment are there?

Let's list them here, roughly in order based on the seriousness of the cancer, for example, whether it's spread outside the prostate gland, and how far.

- Watchful waiting
- External-beam radiation
- Seed implantation radiation
- Surgery—with or without radiation
- Hormones

Am I likely to need chemotherapy?

For now, the medical community says that chemotherapy doesn't work very well on prostate cancer. As new medications and new research emerge, that may change, but you can rest assured that chemo is not one of the treatments you are likely to undergo. See the Learning section of Day Seven for more about this.

What are the side effects I might have from any of the usual treatments?

The most common physical side effects from surgery and radiation are impotence and incontinence, though only about 30 percent of men experience these. These may or may not be permanent. You might also have some diarrhea, blood in your urine, and pain when ejaculating or urinating. The latter symptoms would most likely go away shortly after your treatment.

With more serious cancers that need hormones or painkillers, there may be other side effects. For instance, if your cancer requires **estrogen**, you may show some growth in the size of your breasts, or you may lose some pubic hair. When the hormone treatment ends, these changes will probably return to normal.

But I might become impotent . . . forever?

If you become impotent, either partially or totally, because of treatment, the possibility of reversing the condition to the prior state of affairs is low. You can use drugs now on the market (and more are likely to appear) that can increase blood flow to your penis (this flow is necessary for an erection), and there are both mechanical and surgical options—discussed in Week Four—which have pluses and minuses for this condition.

What about incontinence?

The improvements in all the treatments for prostate cancer make it less and less likely that you will become incontinent, but with surgery it's still fairly high. The chance of reversing such a condition is very much dependent on an individual's physiological configuration in the areas surrounding his prostate, and on the particular treatment he received. In other words, you're unlikely to experience the condition unless you have surgery, but we can't gauge at this time whether, if you do have it following surgery, you'll have to learn to live with some degree of incontinence for the rest of your life.

What kind of pain is associated with the disease or its treatment?

The good news is that, for most men with prostate cancer these days, the disease will not have progressed to the point where painful measures have to be taken (apart from perhaps a brief period of recovery from surgery), nor will you have painful symptoms.

The disease itself has almost no pain in its early and middle stages. Only when it has metastasized is it likely that you will be in some pain, as other areas of the body are attacked by the cancer.

Having said that, these days almost all pain can be handled by a variety of methods, including hormone treatments and radiation to shrink the tumor. In addition, there are powerful and safe analgesics that work very well.

The above applies to physical pain. There is emotional pain that may accompany prostate cancer, including embarrassment, shame, anxiety, and depression. In later chapters, I'll discuss coping mechanisms to deal with these.

What medical advances may we look forward to?

There are at least five or six different ways to treat prostate cancer at the present time, and more are in the pipeline. Due in part to the efforts of Michael Milken (aka the "junk bond king") who had serious prostate cancer himself, money has been flowing into the research efforts on this disease in increasing amounts. Also, numerous trial studies are underway to evaluate everything from the value of present diagnostic tools like the PSA test to what life expectancy various treatment regimens may yield. See the Learning section of Month Nine and Month Eleven.

IN A SENTENCE:

There are numerous ways to live with this cancer, and researchers are seeking more solutions.

DAY 7

living

Radiation

WHEN ROENTGEN discovered the X-ray, and Madame Curie discovered **radium**, no one could possibly have had any notion of how useful and also how dangerous both of these could be. Mme. Curie died from radium poisoning. The fact is, too much of it can kill you and just the right amount can be used to treat you.

What is radiation?

Radiation is a form of energy emitted in the form of waves or particles. The medical term *radiation* means beams from high-powered X-rays or from radioactive material. Unless you ask, you won't really know which form is being used. So, ask.

With either, the best way to get the proper dose is to focus upon a very limited area that needs treatment. This allows a narrow beam to be aimed at just that area. Early stages of prostate cancer are, therefore, ideal for these penetrating rays. If a tumor is completely encapsulated within the gland, pinpoint radiation can be extremely useful in eliminating the cancerous cells.

Over the years, this kind of radiation has grown in usage and in sophistication, as both an alternative and an additive to surgery. It's an alternative when the cancer is very limited in scope, and an additive when surgery cannot guarantee to have found all the malignant cells. This form of treatment has led to other ideas about the use of radioactive materials (which we'll get to in the next chapter).

Radiation doesn't work when cancer has spread to the lymph nodes, because you can't go around blasting all your nodes with rays. That would be dangerous. But if you have large self-contained tumors that have metastasized from your prostate, those can also be attacked with **external-beam radiation** treatment. Thus, the NCI says that external-beam radiation is often used to treat Stage III cancers as well—before surgery, after, or as a stand-alone treatment.

The procedure for getting just the right amount of X-rays to a Stage III tumor via external beam radiation equipment is technically complex and requires a great deal of expertise. If you opt for that kind of radiation, it is imperative that you receive treatment at a facility that does a lot of this kind of therapy and has a good reputation.

For the moment, however, let's assume that the cancer we're talking about is a Stage I or II cancer, with a moderate Gleason score. Your oncologist has the equipment available and tells you that he thinks a number of weeks of daily high-energy X-ray beams can shrink your tumor and give you what he actually calls "a cure." In other words, so sure is he that this will work he doesn't even say "remission."

Getting ready

Here's what the technicians and medical personnel will do in order to make sure the treatment hits the right spots and doesn't hit the wrong ones.

First, you will have a CAT scan. Even if you've had one to diagnose your cancer, you may need to get a second one to pinpoint where the X-rays are needed, and to plot the path to them in a computer formula.

Second, you will lie on the same table on which you will get the radiation and be fitted for a plastic mold. This is done to make sure that, when you're receiving radiation, you're in exactly the same position, time after time. The technicians will use their computerized map to find the spots through which radiation must enter your body; they will put a wet plastic mass on your entire backside, one that dries very quickly, spreading it to cover you from one side to the other, from your midback to your midthighs.

After it dries, they will attach clasps that clamp the mold to the table. Every time you lie down, this mold will be placed on you to guarantee as closely as possible that you are lying in the same spot, and that you receive exactly the same treatment in exactly the same locations inside you.

During the treatment itself, the X-ray machine makes a complete circle around you, so that its beams are penetrating your tumor(s) from every angle. But the computerized map is designed to see that those rays avoid crucial organs (liver, kidney, etc.), as well as veins, nerves, and other parts of the body that you do not want treated. As you can imagine, this is possible only to a certain degree. If you want the tumor gone, you have to allow some degree of leeway on where the beams go.

However, this particular pinpoint technology is far better than the earlier versions of the machines, which sent powerful X-rays into a body without the kind of microscopic limits available in the new equipment. Again, when you are searching for a place to get treated, you would do well to ask if they have the latest equipment.

My experiences with radiation

I found that the worst part of this treatment was the waiting. I would get an appointment to arrive at the hospital every weekday for approximately seven weeks, often at different times of day. (That's right, thirty-five days: it's a long treatment period!) I would go to the waiting room and wait. And wait. That's because a lot of people were getting treated. It's also because there were not many such machines in any hospital. And it's because occasionally a machine malfunctioned and needed to be taken out of service; no one—especially yourself—wants to be treated by a machine unless it's up and running perfectly!

An attendant would eventually call and tell me to change into a gown. I went to a dressing room, changed, and then followed the attendant to my treatment facility. This was a largish room with a huge piece of equipment, surrounded by lead-lined doors.

Lying facedown on the table, the plastic mold was fitted over my waist and buttocks. It was clamped down. The technicians left the room. Buzzing started (the first time it's very startling), and I received a few minutes of rays. That's it. It was over until the next day.

Benefits

Radiation will blast away the cancer, shrinking and eventually removing it, as if by an invisible eraser. As it decreases and eliminates the areas of malignancy, your PSA will probably drop. Whether this treatment will add years to your life is still under study, just as it is with surgery.

Side effects

When radiation is used as an adjunct to surgery, it is not as pinpointed as in the above case. That is because already your prostate and some attached vessels have been removed. The radiation is intended to make sure that any cancerous cells that have not been caught by surgery will be destroyed. Since those cells are not visible (or they would have been removed by the surgeon), the radiation has to be somewhat wider in nature, though again your doctors will do everything they can to make sure your other organs are not damaged.

Because the radiation beam passes through normal tissues—the rectum, the bladder, the intestines—on its way to the prostate, it kills some healthy cells. Radiation to the rectum often causes diarrhea, but the diarrhea usually clears up when treatment is over. And there are some other side effects.

Fatigue

Of all the side effects noticed by cancer patients during and after radiation, fatigue is the most discussed. Depending on the length and strength and kind of radiation, it crops up in most cases.[1]

According to experts, this kind of exhaustion can have all sorts of causes, and can happen without radiation, and in fact without any treatment at all, which makes dealing with it complicated. This is as good a place to deal with the general topic of exhaustion as anywhere in the book, since most patients attribute their fatigue to the radiation they've received.

It often starts with the diagnosis of prostate cancer, and that's clearly a psychological reaction. But sometimes it doesn't begin—this lethargy, tiredness, weakness—until you've begun radiation treatment. Is this because you know you're supposed to get tired from radiation? Is it because the radiation kills healthy cells as well as malignant ones?

Or is it because there are factors at work that science hasn't explained yet? From different doctors, you'll get all three explanations—and more!

One of the annoying things about fatigue during radiation is that you are being made to feel sicker just at the time when you had hoped the treatment was working. If you're of a positive nature, you can use the exhaustion as a sign that treatment is doing its job, and look forward to the end of your radiation regimen. If you're of a negative nature, however, this exhaustion— which can keep some men from going to work, or playing golf, or engaging with friends and family—is just one more upsetting factor in an already upsetting sequence of events. You may feel you are getting worse, instead of being healed. You may not take as good care of other aspects of your health as you should during this time, by being too tired to do your usual workout or to eat properly if it involves too much food preparation or going out. And being tired makes decision making difficult, too.

Then, there are the very practical matters. You may wonder: how can I make a living if I'm tired all the time? How can I keep up my house, take care of my family? If someone, such as your partner, takes over for you, it may cause you to feel helpless rather than helped. All in all, feeling fatigued may result in your feeling depressed, which only serves to exacerbate the exhaustion.

Making diagnosis of fatigue more difficult is the fact that the opposite may be happening: depression is often accompanied by exhaustion. The wish to lie down and nap, or to sleep for hours and hours can be a result of psychological problems, as well as nutritional deficiencies, as well as "dying cells."

If resting doesn't relieve your symptoms—and there's nothing wrong with naps!—then it's worth talking to your doctor(s) about this problem.

Because the causes are so complex, doctors just don't know which factors are responsible for exhaustion in individual men. Here is what they do know:

○ While fatigue may indicate that your cancer is progressing, it is not generally one of the symptoms of prostate cancer.
○ Some fatigue may be due to the fact that your body needs to repair cells damaged by treatment.
○ While fatigue might indicate that the cancer has spread, for the

75 percent of men with contained tumors, it is unlikely that all fatigue is a sign of spreading tumors.

O While some fatigue comes from the *stress* of having prostate cancer, because you are fighting the disease on many fronts (physical, psychological, spiritual), its prevalence as radiation progresses makes it doubtful that all fatigue is a result of such stress.

O If you are taking drugs to combat your anxiety or depression, you're likely to be tired for a while, but that side effect usually reverses itself while the fatigue from prostate cancer treatment by such methods as radiation gets worse for most men for a while—until some time after treatment ceases.

O As you undergo treatment, your hormonal balance may change; your metabolism may change; you may have difficulty sleeping because of anxiety. You may not get enough exercise. Or, you may have some other health problem.

You may not be aware of all these factors in your life because you're concentrating on your cancer. But all these factors, plus many more, can make you tired.

Still, the unknowns in the matter of fatigue during radiation outweigh the knowns. My radiation oncologist said to me, "We just don't know," and left it at that.

After surgery, fatigue is likely because any major operation will leave patients—especially older ones—feeling tired. Muscles begin to atrophy if they are not used for even a few days of bed rest; your body may be sapped of sufficient nutrients until you are back to eating as usual again; and the hospital experience itself may be stressful or depressing.

With hormone therapy (for Stage III and IV patients), which we'll get to in the following chapter, exhaustion may be one side effect of having the chemistry of your body altered by the drugs.

Other side effects

Fatigue usually goes away after radiation, but the treatment can also cause a variety of long-term problems. These include proctitis (inflammation of the rectum), with bleeding and bowel problems such as diarrhea; and cystitis (inflammation of the bladder), leading to problems with urination.

Some men become incontinent, though fewer with radiation than with surgery. And some become impotent.

Again, having the best hospital with the best equipment can reduce the problems you may encounter with radiation therapy.

IN A SENTENCE:

For certain kinds of cancer, beam radiation can find a tumor and blast it away.

learning

Why Not Chemotherapy?

YOU MAY be wondering why I don't list chemotherapy as an option. Perhaps you know or have read about people who have undergone this treatment for other forms of cancer.

What is chemotherapy?

Chemotherapy essentially fights fire with fire: it introduces measured amounts of poisonous chemicals into a person's body—low enough not to kill the person, but high enough to kill the cancer. This effect was discovered by accident during World War II, when an explosion that released mustard gas produced effects that scientists realized could shrink or eliminate systemwide malignancies, such as those within bones or in the lymph system. The drugs developed since that time all work on that same principle: somehow, they "kill" the cancerous cells (which multiply more rapidly than do normal cells) by interfering with their ability to reproduce.

Why prostate cancer is different

Chemotherapy works best on tumors that grow quickly. However, prostate cancer cells grow slowly (with some exceptions, which I'll get to), so that in Stages I through III of most prostate cancers, chemotherapy turns out to be of no use whatsoever. The amount of chemo used to efficiently attack such cancers would have to be so strong that they would damage your normal cells, too.

Chemo for stage IV prostate cancer

In Stage IV, when prostate cancer has metastasized into other areas of the body and *is* progressing more speedily, chemotherapy is one possible treatment, but has not yet been shown to be the best kind for this particular kind of cancer.

The best way of slowing down the growth or spread of even advanced prostate cancer, and of shrinking the tumors, still remains hormone therapy. However, chemotherapy is in the process of being tested in these cases, and has demonstrated a limited effect on tumor growth and pain. According to the American Cancer Society, "Although it may slow tumor growth and reduce pain, [chemotherapy] has had limited success for the treatment of advanced disease." The NCI is even more downbeat: "To date, no evidence indicates that chemotherapy prolongs survival."

The NCI continues to research this area and will report regularly on whether chemo works.

For those few advanced patients who may be advised to try chemotherapy, here are a few words about what to expect.

How is chemotherapy administered?

For decades, chemotherapy was traditionally an in-hospital process, in which patients reported for multiple sessions on a fixed schedule and to receive intravenous administration of the anticancer drug. More recently, chemo has been given by mouth or by injection, which doesn't eliminate the multiple sessions but at least speeds up the treatment per session.

These are very strong medications and need to be administered at regular intervals to be effective. This demands dedication on the part of the patient to see the treatment through. You can't skip appointments, or skip a dose and then just take two pills later.

Side effects

Because the drugs kill not just cancer cells but also other quick-growing cells, such as those for hair or mucosal cells in your digestive system, they can have an overall negative effect on many systems of the body. It used to be said that the "cure is worse than the disease." But recent developments have lowered the overall poisonous character of chemotherapy, made it easier to administer and its side effects less villainous.

Common side effects may include:

○ Anemia
○ Reduced ability of the blood to clot
○ Mouth sores
○ Increased likelihood of developing infections
○ Loss of appetite
○ Nausea or vomiting
○ Diarrhea
○ Weight loss
○ Exhaustion
○ Hair loss

No wonder chemotherapy is used only when considered necessary and valuable. But, as I said, in just the last few years valuable strides have been made in reducing these side effects.

How to counteract the effects of chemo

The hair loss associated with chemotherapy may be a moot point for many men, but for those for whom it is not, rest assured that once chemo treatments end, your hair follicles will recover and replenish what has been lost.

Far more important is to make sure your nutritional needs continue to be satisfied during the weeks of therapy. You need a strong body to fight cancer, and also to sustain the rigors of the chemo substances themselves. Whether you may have simply lost your appetite or have actually experienced vomiting or diarrhea, chances are that you have not only been losing weight but have developed vitamin and mineral deficiencies and dehydration. It may be undernourishment that is triggering other side effects you think are being caused directly by the chemo, such as cracked lips.

Your oncological team may not be monitoring your diet or may not be knowledgeable about nutrition, so it is vital that you bring up the subject with your primary care physician, even if you have been overweight and don't mind losing a few pounds. At the very least, he should take a simple blood test to determine what vitamin and mineral deficiencies or other chemical imbalances may have kicked in since your treatment began. And he may send you to a nutritionist, who will analyze what your body needs not only to regain its nutrient balance, but build up your strength. She will likely recommend specific supplements, as well as a diet high in low-fat proteins, fiber, vitamins A, B-complex, and C, all of which boost your body's defense system.

Exercise is another valuable countermeasure to the destructiveness of your treatment. While you may feel too tired to even think about it, the fact is that slight to moderate exercise during this period will actually *give* you more energy. If you are physically active, you are also less likely to experience nausea or other digestive upsets, by the diversion of some of the blood from your abdomen into the muscles of your limbs (which of course is also very good for your limbs). And don't forget the psychological boost you can get from exercise. As you may know from vigorous workouts, it can be a terrific stress-reducer. What may begin as forcing yourself to take a daily walk outdoors or swim at a gym may become a high point of your day, as it enables you to forget about your treatment and lose yourself in how good your body feels just then.

Overall, maintaining as normal a life as possible during treatment is vital to your well-being. This is no time to turn your back on the richness of your life. So, work around your therapy schedule to continue to include activities you enjoy, family, and friends. Don't use the regimen as an excuse to retreat from either the world or yourself.

Is chemotherapy for you?

Comfort level is all important when patients are in the advanced stages of any disease, and the medical profession is well aware that comfort (i.e., quality of life) can be almost as important to a cancer patient in advanced stages as whether he or she will survive. If your oncologist wishes to try it but you find its potential side effects off-putting, it is your right to refuse this treatment. And if you try chemo, and it makes you feel truly terrible, you have every right to opt out of continuing with the therapy.

For those who wish to forge ahead regardless of its unknown success rate and possible side effects—more power to you! The benefits of less pain and/or an extended life may, in your case, be well worth dealing with chemo.

IN A SENTENCE:

> *Although chemotherapy is not effective in Stage I through III prostate cancers, Stage IV patients may eventually find it beneficial.*

FIRST-WEEK MILESTONE

Here's what I covered in this book so far. If you have trouble remembering something, you can always use the index to find it again, but you also have this milestone box to come back to.

○ YOU'VE LEARNED THE BASIC NATURE OF PROSTATE CANCER, AND HOW YOU HAPPEN TO HAVE IT.

○ YOU'VE SEEN THAT IT IS NOT NECESSARY TO PANIC; YOU CAN PLAN AHEAD SLOWLY.

○ YOU'VE LEARNED THAT THERE ARE SEVERAL DEGREES OF PROSTATE CANCER AND HOW THEY MAY BE TREATED.

○ YOU'VE LEARNED HOW IMPORTANT IT IS TO GET A SECOND OPINION AND TO LOOK FOR THE BEST DOCTOR AND HOSPITAL IN WHICH TO GET TREATED.

○ YOU'VE LEARNED ABOUT THE CONCEPT OF "WATCHFUL WAITING" AS AN ACTUAL TREATMENT. ONE THAT MIGHT WORK FOR YOU AS CONTRASTED WITH OTHER MORE ACTIVE TREATMENTS.

○ YOU'VE BECOME ACQUAINTED WITH SOME OF THE CONTROVERSY SURROUNDING PROSTATE CANCER SCREENING AND TREATMENT.

Seed Implantation and Hormone Therapy

Seed implantation

Only about ten years ago, the treatment of prostate cancer was in its infancy. It has come a very long way since then. One of the more recent treatments that has found its way into practice (many more proposed treatments are still being tested in clinical trials) is seed implantation. This is the use of tiny slivers of radioactive material that are inserted into the prostate through the wall of your rectum. The radiation is relatively short-term in its power, but it lasts long enough to attack the cancerous cells.

The technical term for this treatment is brachytherapy. It can be done while you're an outpatient, takes about two hours, and is, by now, a fairly routine procedure in many hospitals, big and even medium-size.

Because the radiation is administered very close to your cancerous cells (a special computer program plus a CAT scan helps the technicians place the seeds), you may avoid damage to other organs and vessels. In this way, impotence and incontinence may be partially sidestepped—though there is no guarantee that they will not result from this.

Since the seeds—made from radioactive palladium or iodine—lose their radioactivity after a few weeks, they are safe to leave in the prostate.

An alternative method is known as temporary brachytherapy. It involves the placement of several tiny plastic catheters into the prostate, wherever cancer cells have been detected. A highly radioactive seed is pushed through each catheter by a computer-controlled device. It is left in for a specified amount of time, depending on the location of the catheter. For instance, a seed that is positioned near the urethra or sensitive nerves is pulled out sooner than one inserted into the center of the prostate. The temporary method has some psychological and physiological benefits over the implantation method, since no seeds are left in the patient's body after the catheters are withdrawn.

With the permanent implantation method, patients are cautioned not to have sex for some months after receiving the treatment, since occasionally a seed has been known to migrate into a channel that leads into the penis, and thus may be ejected accidentally during ejaculation into a woman's vagina, where stray radiation is to be avoided at all costs.

But, aside from the abstention issue, which is only temporary and at worst frustrating, it is assumed that there are no dangerous side effects from the radiation. It is important to point out, however, that brachytherapy is new enough in the field that really good long-term analyses have not been made. Still, researchers feel that surgery, external beam radiation, and seed implantation—when used properly for the right kind of tumor configuration—are equally effective.

Benefits

Seed implantation is best used for Stage I or II prostate cancer, where the disease is presumed not to have spread into other organs or into the lymph system. It is not useful for especially large tumors.

Seed implantation costs less than other kinds of radiation (or surgery, obviously), and imposes much less of a time demand on patients. Not having to go to the hospital daily for seven weeks is a definite advantage.

Possible problems

While the benefits are great, there are those who would not put radioactive seeds in their body for anything in the world. Anxiety over this issue can make some men hesitant to even consider seed implantation.

In addition, there is no promise that incontinence or impotence will not occur, though the risks are less than with other treatment modalities. Prostatitis may occur. And some minor pain may result from the insertion of the seeds themselves.

Hormone therapy

Hormone therapy is primarily used with a Stage IV or Stage III cancer. These cancers are not controlled by radiation or seed implantation therapy because the malignant cells have invaded other tissues and organs of the body. These cancers cannot, at this time, be cured. They can be slowed down and, clearly, you and your oncologists will want to cripple the growth of the spreading malignancy as much as you can. The slower the growth of the cells, the longer before bone cancer causes pain, and so the longer you can live relatively comfortably with even these kinds of cancer.

Hormones used for this purpose deprive the cancerous cells of male hormones, such as testosterone. Male hormones help cancer cells grow. Doctors use the term "hormonal therapy" to apply to the use of drugs, and to even, in some cases, the surgical removal of the source of testosterone—the testicles.

One of the drugs used in hormone therapy is estrogen, the female counterpart of testosterone. Estrogen is responsible for many of a woman's sexual characteristics. Estrogen counters the testosterone in the man's body and slows growth of prostate cancer cells.

In addition, hormones have been used prior to prostate surgery to shrink tumors, so less tissue needs to be removed. I believe that was the case with Rudy Giuliani, New York's former mayor, who made his treatment public as a service to men who were not aware of the disease or were ashamed to talk about it.

Pain control

Hormone therapy has another, very important use. For Stage IV cancer, where the malignancy has spread into other organs and tissues, or into the bones, hormone therapy can cut down on the discomfort and pain associated with metastasizing cancer. In conjunction with pain medication, a man's life can be made more comfortable with the use of hormone therapy, even if he has Stage IV prostate cancer.

New studies are also looking at whether hormone therapy might be used to stop prostate cancer before it spreads, as an alternative or adjunct to radiation. For more on this, Month Nine.

Cutting out the source of testosterone

The decision to surgically castrate a patient or to use drugs containing estrogen is one that a doctor will take very seriously—as will you—and will depend on where the cancer is, how far it has spread, and other deeply technical considerations. (For those whose testicles are removed, it may be some comfort to know that the scrotum is not eliminated or diminished, and that **prosthetic** testes can be inserted into it.)

Hormones other than estrogen can be used. One kind, injected into the patient, actually signals the brain to keep the testes from producing male hormones. And many more experiments with hormones are in the pipeline.[1]

The cons of hormone therapy

While cutting off the production of testosterone works very well to shrink tumors, it also produces side effects. Sexual arousal can be diminished; men can actually experience female menopausal symptoms, such as hot flashes; and—with the use of estrogen—a man's breasts can become enlarged. (Estrogen is what is used when men wish to change gender; it produces some of the female sexual characteristics that they want to have.) Other possible side effects are fever, chill, and fatigue. For men to whom these adverse side effects are physically unpleasant and psychologically disturbing, the discontinuation of the drugs will reverse the effects.

For men with early (Stage I or II) cancer, these potential side effects may not be worth it, but what about men with Stage III or IV, where pain and the spread of the malignancy are too important to ignore? Recent studies have shown that hormone therapy for six months is as effective as what had been the most current practice, which was to use the hormones for up to three years.[2] A briefer treatment period will prove a winning notion for the future, since, aside from the side effects I've mentioned, prolonged use of hormones can cause heart or stroke problems in men.

There's another caveat to consider: Typically, the hormone-fueled respite from cell growth does not last. For a variety of reasons, the effect of the hormones diminishes, and cancerous cells begin to grow again after two or three years. So, prostate cancer patients who opt for hormone therapy will enjoy only limited success with this method. Scientists are presently experimenting with other hormones that may be used to contain a resurgence of a malignancy already treated with hormones.

IN A SENTENCE:

> *Seed implantation and hormone therapy are exciting new treatments that bear both investigation and caution.*

learning

Complementary Medicine

In addition to hormone therapy, "Milken decided to change his diet radically to one virtually devoid of fat. As a supplement to Western medicine, he added meditation, sesame-oil massages, aromatherapy, and yoga. . . . He starts each morning with a shake—a mix of antioxidants including brewed green tea, lemon zest, vitamin E, and a micronutrient called genistein that is found in some soybeans.—*Fortune* magazine, November 2004

WHAT IS often called mainstream (or Western or conventional) medicine is not the only type of treatment available to people with a serious illness. More and more people are seeking care that reaches beyond mainstream medicine to what is loosely called **alternative medicine**. For instance, while most American physicians do not usually suggest medications that have not been approved by the Food and Drug Administration (FDA), alternative practitioners may offer herbs or other kinds of drugs or treatments that have not been so approved.

Complementary medicine is on the march

As time progresses, many within the American medical system are finding it useful to erase some of those boundaries between mainstream care and the arena of alternative medicine. The use of both kinds of approaches—one that treats the body through mainstream approaches, the other treating not only the body but the mind and spirit as well, has many attractions.

The coordinated use of both mainstream and alternative medicine is called complementary medicine; but to accommodate those to whom this term is new, in common usage is the term **Complementary and Alternative Medicine (CAM)** to refer to the practices, health-care systems, and products that are *not* presently considered to be part of mainstream medicine.

For the most part, these practices have been borrowed from India, China, and other parts of the world where they were in use long before Western medicine reached those countries. These practices and medicines (many taken from plant and animal life, rather than produced in a lab) were developed over a long period of time and refined to a point where those societies gained confidence in their efficacy. Western scientists, doubtful at first, have shown increasing interest in learning from the East, and have begun incorporating some of the practices and substances into their work. So it is that **acupuncture**, chiropractic, Qi Gong, herbal medicine, and other disciplines have been licensed in the United States, England, and elsewhere in Europe; in some cases, they are even paid for by insurance companies.

Aromatherapy, therapeutic massage, meditation, spiritual practices, and many more are now part of the panoply of treatments available to those with diseases or illness. In fact, a major cancer center, such as Memorial Sloan-Kettering in New York City, will offer workshops in a wide variety of these, under titles like "Touch therapies" (Reiki, shiatsu, aromatherapy), "Mind-body Therapies" (meditation, guided imagery, self-hypnosis), "Movement and Fitness" (aerobics, Qi Gong, the Alexander technique, and many more), and "Nutritional Counseling."

The use of CAM has grown rapidly in the United States in recent years. According to the National Institutes of Health's (NIH) Center on CAM, a survey reveals that more than 60 percent of doctors from a wide range of specialties have recommended alternative therapies to their patients at least once. Half of the doctors in that study reported using alternative therapies themselves.

Seventy-five out of 117 U.S. medical schools now offer elective courses in CAM or include CAM topics in required courses.

However, the actual use of CAM by patients may not be nearly as widespread as the above statistics would imply. One journal reported that fewer than one-third of the adults in the United States have used CAM therapies as frequently as once a year.[3]

Just to confuse things more, one could look at the financial side of CAM in America. According to one Web site, a few years ago "Americans spent $13.7 billion on 425 million visits to alternative practitioners, compared with $12.8 billion on 385 million visits to primary care **allopathic** physicians."[4]

Advocates of CAM say that mainstream medicine very often does not provide relief from such serious diseases as cancer, and that to withhold CAM from patients for whom other treatment is not sufficient, is to deny hope and possible ease of their diseases. Many patients report that some forms of CAM help to reduce stress. And, according to the NIH center, some people use CAM not only because they are dissatisfied with conventional medicine, but because these health care alternatives mirror their own values, beliefs, and philosophical orientations toward health and life.

On the other hand, the field is still controversial. Some physicians, trained for years in mainstream medicine, do not believe in the benefit of alternative practices. While they do not necessarily frown on their patients' use of Asian herbs or acupuncture or other therapies, they themselves want demonstrable proof that this kind of medicine can actually be effective. Some claim that there is even evidence that some of the remedies can actually do harm, or at least interfere with the value of conventional, tested medicines.

One of the reasons for doubt on the part of mainstream medical practitioners is the long history of not only fraudulent claims for what are in other ways legitimate CAM therapies but crazes that have involved patients trying to get cures from totally baseless alternative medications or from charlatans offering "miracles."

In addition, while some alternative medications or practices may be helpful under some circumstances, under others the combination of herbs with prescription medications has turned out to be either harmful or contraindicated.

The case of the inside of peach pits—called Amygdalin or Laetrile—is famous in the annals of alternative medicine. Laetrile was supposed to be a cure for cancer. The ACS called it a hoax but hundreds of patients went to Mexico to get the drug, to save themselves from otherwise terminal cancer. Hope, money, and lives went down the drain.

Because of this kind of controversy, various organizations have begun to try to find out whether CAM provides benefits that can be proven.

In 1998, Congress established the National Center for Complementary and Alternative Medicine (NCCAM), with the mandate to encourage and develop research on CAM. While the U.S. government is interested in alternative forms of treatment, NCCAM wants to make sure that the studies it supports are looking at CAM in a rigorously scientific manner. It does not willy-nilly advocate alternative therapies but, rather, asks for double-blind studies and all the other hallmarks of good research to determine their effectiveness and safety.

Additionally, in 2000, a presidential commission on CAM was set up to establish policy to assure the effectiveness of CAM medications and treatments, as well as the dissemination of information about CAM, and approval and education of CAM practitioners.

Most scientists and researchers in the U.S. medical establishment want to keep a rigorous approach to the analysis of all medicines and medical practices. They do not want to accept new ones—especially herbs and other medications—which may have been used for centuries, but where only **anecdotal evidence** exists to prove their safety and value.

For that reason, NCI and NCCAM are financing clinical trials to study how CAM can be used for various types of cancer or the side effects of its conventional treatments.[5]

What CAM therapies are useful for prostate cancer?

One study showed that about two-thirds of patients in its group had used some form of CAM for their type of cancer, but since this could include as diverse a collection of therapies as chiropractic, acupuncture, or aromatherapy, it is hard to tell what that study actually means in terms of the huge number of medicines and practices that fall under CAM. We do not yet have conclusive evidence concerning any specific therapy or drug.

We need to divide the issue into two parts:

1. What CAM therapies work to make patients' lives more pleasant (for instance, reduce pain or nausea)?
2. Which therapies seem to work to reduce tumors?

As long ago as 1997, the National Institutes of Health said it had found that acupuncture was useful in controlling pain from surgery, as well as some nausea from chemotherapy, but as to killing malignant cells, acupuncture has no effect whatsoever.

What's being studied now?

According to NCCAM and NCI, there are clinical trials to see if:

○ Acupuncture can reduce symptoms of advanced colorectal cancer.
○ Shark cartilage makes chemotherapy more effective in patients with some forms of lung cancer.
○ Some forms of massage will help fight exhaustion that comes from certain cancers.
○ Mistletoe extract helps when combined with chemotherapy in certain cancers.

There are a variety of Web sites on which the NCI and its associated divisions list clinical trials. See "Other Resources" at the end of this book for those locations.

What CAM therapies are being used on prostate cancer?

While it is known that many prostate cancer patients use dietary supplements or change their eating habits, it is not clear from any current surveys how many explore such CAM therapies as herbal medicines, meditation, acupuncture, etc.

So far, most studies involve treatment of those who already have prostate cancer; however, NCCAM and other groups are in the middle of several clinical trials looking at some possible preventive strategies, for instance:

○ The mineral selenium is being tested for possible preventive effects in what's called The Selenium and Vitamin E Cancer Prevention Trial (SELECT).
○ Lycopene, an **antioxidant** commonly found in tomatoes and tomato-based products, is also being studied. According to the NCI, a trial at Northwestern University is inquiring whether tomato oil with a high concentration of lycopene might impede the development of

some forms of prostate cancer. Lycopene usage in normal diets has been correlated already in some studies with a lower rate of cancer in some people. According to a press release from Northwestern University and the NCI, "Research has shown an over 20 percent reduced risk for developing prostate cancer in men who ate more cooked tomato products, such as tomato sauce. Additional studies showed that cooking tomatoes and eating them with oil substantially increases the bioavailability of lycopene."[6]

What should patients do when using or considering complementary and alternative therapies?

According to NCCAM, "Cancer patients using or considering complementary or alternative therapy should discuss this decision with their doctor or nurse, as they would any therapeutic approach. Some complementary and alternative therapies may interfere with standard treatment or may be harmful when used with conventional treatment. It is also a good idea to become informed about the therapy, including whether the results of scientific studies support the claims that are made for it."

When considering CAM therapies, ask your doctor:

○ What benefits can be expected from this therapy?
○ What are the risks associated with this therapy?
○ Do the known benefits outweigh the risks?
○ What side effects can be expected?
○ Will the therapy interfere with conventional treatment?
○ Is this therapy part of a clinical trial? If so, who is sponsoring the trial?
○ Will the therapy be covered by health insurance?

Where can I go for further information?

See "Other Resources" at the end of this book.

IN A SENTENCE:

> *Complementary and alternative medicine is gaining some legitimacy in the war against cancer.*

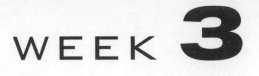

WEEK 3

living

Telling Family, Friends, and Colleagues

> When I saw the look on my wife's face, I knew that how I was going to have to deal with my cancer was nothing compared to how she was going to deal with it. I had never seen such pain in her face. And it was me causing it.—MARVIN N., diagnosed with Stage II prostate cancer

> When he told me he had prostate cancer, I felt a pain right here—in my chest—that wasn't going to go away. I just knew that. It would be there forever.—GEORGIA N.

YOUR FAMILY, friends, and colleagues can only imagine what you're going through. And you may not be able to tell them that you're not as frightened as they think you are . . . or that you're more frightened. They may think your contracting cancer is the worst thing that can possibly happen to you—and to them. It's bad enough to be suffering from this disease yourself, but now they are suffering, too.

As this process winds its course, you will learn things about your wife, your children, and yourself. As one man put it: "Marriage is redefined."

My wife's reaction

My wife, Susan, is compassionate. She's a psychotherapist. She listens, then she asks questions; she knows about stress and anxiety and depression. She rescues people—not dramatically, like Wonder Woman, not for forever, but for now, which is often enough.

We talk—often late at night—about how she tries to find her way through the maze of feelings and problems that she has to face daily because her patients are facing them: the myriad attacks on the human spirit. But neither of us ever expected her to have to deal with my depression and anxiety when I got prostate cancer ten years after I thought lymphoma was the last I would ever see of a malignant cell.

I realized how different things were when I came home after my third day of radiation and found her at the table, looking very sad. "What's wrong?" I asked, casually. She smiled wanly, and said, "My husband has cancer."

To tell the truth, I was a little taken back. I had thought that the impact of this disease would all be on me. That the sorrow would be mine. That love and attention and care would be showered upon me. Now, I suddenly saw that things were not quite that simple. She was in very real pain, as well.

How cancer affects loved ones

While you are struggling with your mortality, you need to look at the larger picture: your wife or partner is, too. (Though this applies equally to male partners, I hope they will forgive me if I use the term "she" here.) You may be anxious, but so may she. You may feel angry, but so may she. Only *she* may not be "allowed" to express it—because of her own self-control, or perhaps because you are refusing to listen. Because it would look as if she is unsupportive. Or because it would be "selfish" of her to express such feelings when she's not the one in danger.

Only she *is* in danger. She's in danger of losing—or at least believes she's in danger of losing—someone she cares about deeply. Her entire image of your shared future together has been thrown out of focus, and she's scrambling to make sense of it.

If you aren't teamed up with someone, don't think that leaves you out of this chapter. Friends, colleagues, and other relatives can feel the impact of your cancer just as much as wives or partners.

So let's get on with three lessons:

1. Your acceptance of others' fear and pain.
2. Their learning how to deal with your cancer.
3. Deciding whom to tell outside your most intimate circle.

Fear and pain

Most wives expect, deep down, that their husbands will die first. In our society—where women generally marry someone older than themselves—husbands usually do. In addition, there's something about women that gives them a longer life to begin with.

Knowing this is one thing; coming to terms with it is another. That may be one reason why wives are usually better at getting their husbands to go to the doctor when ill: women have more to lose.

If the relationship is a good one and has lasted until you're in your 60s, 70s, or 80s, you can be sure that your wife has thought more than once about what would happen if you became seriously ill and died. But thinking about it is different—far different—from experiencing it. And, unless you've had a chronic disease for a long time, or an accident, or a previous experience with cancer, your wife will be deeply shaken by the news that you have prostate cancer. Especially if she is of an older generation for whom cancer is synonymous with death, she may not hear anything but C-A-N-C-E-R. She may not even recall that, in a women's magazine perhaps, she read that prostate cancer is treatable, or that most men with this disease don't die of it. Even if she knows something about the illness, the fact that *you* have it will be terrifying to her. And it may come out in unexpected ways, if she is not accustomed—and who is ever accustomed—to being afraid for you.

Think of a parent running into the street to pick up a toddler who has strayed into traffic. Rather than cry or tenderly remonstrate with the child, the parent often appears angry. But this is not what the parent is feeling. He/she is feeling intense anxiety: anxiety that the child somehow eluded his/her care; anxiety that the child could have been hurt or killed.

So, too, when your wife feels anxious about your cancer, she may seem irritated or outright angry. About your being late for supper. About not taking out the garbage. About your being tired early in the evening. You, of course, become irritated or upset in turn that she's snapping at you: "Doesn't she know I'm doing my best?" "How can she treat me that way? I'm the one with cancer." And your response is, of course, absolutely correct. Except for one thing: it ignores the fact that your wife desperately wants to turn back the clock to before you were diagnosed, and finds that it's out of her control. Criticism in this case is a means of trying to resume control over at least some things. It's her inability to rid you of the cancer that she is angry at. Not you.

She may experience other reactions that you may need some help interpreting:

Tears

Back in the 1980s, I heard a researcher at the University of Minnesota say that the tears of men and women were chemically different, which might account, he said, for the fact that women cry more often than men. There are other reasons, of course, including men's reluctance to appear weak. Most men don't like to cry in front of others. And a lot of men don't like to have to comfort weeping women.

Well, if you've got cancer, you can bet that your wife or partner is going to cry. Perhaps more often than she used to, and perhaps more than you want her to. Get used to it. It's a sign of how much she cares about you, and how much pain she's in. And keep in mind that needing to cry yourself doesn't make you less of a man.

Blame

This doesn't get expressed very often, but it's definitely something that can fester in the back of someone's mind when illness strikes. The fact is, despite what you and your wife may read or hear about prostate cancer, both you and she are going to eventually wonder if something you did or did not do is responsible for your disease:

- O Did you smoke?
- O Did you drink?
- O Are you overweight?
- O Do you eat too much fatty meat?

○ Did you have sex with someone who could have given it to you?

○ Did you sin against a higher being?

As researchers dig more deeply into the causes of prostate cancer, one or another of these things—barring the last two examples—may actually prove to be a *slight* determinant. But even if they don't, the fact that almost 75 percent of men will eventually get the disease won't deter you and/or your wife from seeking something or someone to blame. This seems to be a very normal fallout of our being logical, wired to believe everything has a cause and effect. Your best weapon against this is for you both to become as knowledgeable as possible about the facts behind the disease. Don't let your emotions be swayed by ignorance.

Sex

In Week Four, I get to the very real problem of impotence: how to accept it as a possibility; how to deal with it as a reality. You and your partner can't help but imagine that your sex life may be hindered, or even halted, by your cancer or the treatment that you will get.

Even if you and your wife have lost some of your prior interest in sex, or don't engage in much sexual activity, I'm going to address this to the millions of men who do take an interest in sex. In short: have you considered your wife's interest in and need for it? The fact that your sex life may diminish temporarily or even permanently as a result of the cancer or its treatment must be addressed. Somehow. Some way. Your physical relationship is an issue that affects and is very important to both of you. It's something to work on together, if impotency asserts itself as an anticipated or genuine problem. I'll get far more into detail about how in Week Four, and again in Month Eight.

What you may be able to discover is (a) talking diplomatically about the issue is helpful; and (b) you will be able to find other means of expressing sexual interest and having sexual pleasure.

You may have tried these tactics before—during other times when relations between you weren't so good, or when you both had grown tired of the way sex was going. But this is a little different. Now your partner's sense of masculinity is threatened because the organs involved with it are under very real physical attack.

This is a time when you both need as much comfort from each other as you can get, and physical comfort is one thing to be explored and shared, not avoided.

When I get to Week Four, I'll talk about what changes may occur, and how you can deal with them as a couple.

A *message to wives and partners*

There is no doubt that men like to feel in charge and powerful.

This prostate cancer business eats away at that. Attacking without any perceivable cause, a tumor does more than change some cells within a small, expendable organ. It can reduce a man's energy, his self-esteem, his sexual drive or ability, and his will to live. All of that reduces his sense of power.

You can feel this. You can sense it. And . . . you can't change it!

If your husband or partner is in mourning for his losses (masculinity, autonomy, sexuality, mortality), he may not want to hear about what you are going through right now. Or you may not want him to know how frightened or sad you are. You may feel that expressing anything negative or doubting appears unloving, or makes you seem weak just when he needs your support.

> I didn't want to hear anything from Franco about all this. I wasn't
> ill. He was. And he kept saying that he knew how upset I was and
> I had the right to be upset, and I didn't want to hear that.

That is a statement from the wife of a man who had prostate cancer. She felt guilty about being angry and fearful and petulant. She felt guilty about being afraid that her husband of forty-two years might die. And she felt doubly guilty, because she knew she didn't have to be afraid: she and her husband had been educated about the fact that his localized prostate cancer wasn't likely to kill him, or even cause him much distress.

After a while, you may find that becoming more knowledgeable about prostate cancer will calm you down and also open the channels to discuss your husband's feelings of loss with him. But perhaps you think you are a terrible person to have *your* feelings. If you feel as if you aren't yourself, if you find yourself more irritable or fearful or tearful than usual, there is every good reason to take yourself to a counselor. Think of it this way: your husband will be happier and you'll be better able to look after him, if you are better able to cope with your own situation.

To other family members

When I got lymphoma, my daughters telephoned me every day. Normally, there are days, even weeks between calls. But at that time, my two daughters called daily. "Hi, Pops. How're you feeling?" or "Hi, Dad. What's new?" There was always some other pretext for the call but I always knew what it was really about: You still there, Pops? You still with us? You making it through this thing?

It made me feel loved. And the funny thing is, they didn't agree on this between them. It wasn't, "You call every day, and so will I, and we'll make him feel loved." No, this was spontaneous, on both their parts. I know; I asked them. Yes, it made me feel very loved and very important to those two young women. They're people I'm glad to know.

The lesson I want to pass on to readers of this book is that this kind of family support is terribly important. You need to keep your communications lines open—not with false sentiment, but with what you are really feeling, and filled with the many aspects of everyday life that are continuing despite the cancer. Don't use the cancer as an excuse not to remember who you are as a whole person.

The thing is, with the exception of this "little problem" of having cancer, I am a healthy man. I'm physically fit and mentally fit and I have to trust that I'm going to land on the right side of the statistics. It's not about denial. I don't minimize the seriousness of this and I'm aware of what's going on, but I'm determined to do two things at once—to act both realistically and optimistically at the same time. One isn't separated from the other. I'm going to do everything possible to fight this disease but, at the same time, I'm not going to let it take over my life. I have a family that I love and I have work that means a lot to me. I'm going to continue to live my life, full tilt, as long as I possibly can.—a cancer patient

What about work?

Having a life-threatening illness in the workplace has its own unique difficulties.

It might be hard to be open with coworkers who are not personal friends. You might be afraid that your quality of work will suffer. And if you tell colleagues, or your employer, they may think your work is suffering, even if it isn't. You may feel uncomfortable with their curiosity about the details of the disease; they may feel uncomfortable with the word "cancer." But they also may take it just as you hoped they would.

> "Oh, my God, I'm so sorry," said my close friend Sherry, at work, when I told her I had prostate cancer. She empathized because she was a good, empathetic person.
>
> I thanked her, and we went on with our business. Aside from occasional questions about how the treatment was going, she never brought it up again. And that was fine by me: she had been thoughtful and caring, and I didn't need to think about it all the time, anyway.—ERNIE G.

Talk to your colleagues

For me, in the workplace, the rule of thumb I discussed about family— talking as openly as possible—still applies. In many people's view, it is the best way to create an environment that is supportive and productive.

> What I found incredibly important was to talk to my colleagues about my diagnosis. As soon as I recovered from the bad news, I talked to everybody in our team. And I felt that I needed to do that because I didn't know what they were going to see. I didn't know if they were going to see a healthy person or someone who was going to decline into a person who is ill. And so I wanted to let them know, to give them permission to talk to me about my disease.
>
> When I did that, they also gave me permission to talk more about it. And from that open dialogue came more support in the

workplace. I think that we need to talk more about illness and death in workplaces everywhere. It's terrible to have this sort of disease or any life-limiting disease and not be able to talk about it to people with whom you work, or with whom you have any kind of enduring commerce.—another patient

"Tapestry of support"

Some years back, a woman named Kathryn "Kit" Meshenberg started recording her thoughts about her virulent cancer. She worked with an organization to create a Web site about her illness. Eventually, she died from the disease, but in the meantime she had educated hundreds or thousands of people, both on and off the Web site. She was not afraid to talk about the disease; not afraid to let people know that she was trying to make her life better, to live fully until the end, whenever that might be.

She coined the term "Tapestry of Support" to refer to those multifaceted support structures that all of us can have, if we reach out: our family, our friends, our health-care providers, our colleagues, our spiritual contacts, our therapists. All can play a role in making us into emotionally and physically more healthy, even as we suffer a serious illness.

> There are different ways that people deal with this. For me, I believe facing a life-threatening illness alone is one of the worst things imaginable so my approach is to line up the best team I can find to support me—a medical team, a spiritual team, different kinds of medicines, family, friends, and colleagues. For me that's part of managing this. You say to yourself—yes, this is a big deal, but I'll be able to do it. And my job is to be as open as possible. If I need somebody's help, my job is to make that clear . . . to say what I need.—KIT MESHENBERG

One of Kit's colleagues—an oncologist—did an interview in which she strove to explain Kit's need to reach out, as well as the enormous benefit it provided to everyone who knew her:

I think, too, that Kit is trying to prove a point for other people in the hospice and palliative care movement as well. She works with me in an organization dedicated to dealing openly and well with life-threatening illness. She makes us think about how we can let this be okay in the workplace. It has become a personal and collegial mission to prove that we can walk the talk that we are teaching everybody. And by golly she does. She is open and honest and it's so smoothly managed it makes me think that vacations and maternity leaves are harder to accommodate than Kit's illness. She's teaching us how to "raise a hand and ask for help" with enormous grace and dignity. She is teaching us how, by supporting her, she can be a full and strong member of the team on whom we rely completely. She has defined the term manager for me, anew. I had no sense of the depth of respect that was due that term until Kit showed me how you can manage an illness, you can manage a team, you can manage life, you can manage all kinds of things, not for the purpose of control, but for the purpose of fulfillment.[1]

Why you may not wish to tell people

When I got cancer for the first time, I had a lot of ambivalence about talking about it. So did my wife. The wish to talk to friends and colleagues was almost unbearable. But, for several reasons, Susan urged me to limit such confidences. For one thing, it wasn't fair to them, she said. For those who cared about me, it would hand them something to worry about, to make them upset. For colleagues, it might make them feel I wasn't capable of carrying on my usual duties, which wasn't true.

In the end, I was willing to go along with silence. Perhaps, I thought, if I didn't tell people, then maybe I wasn't really ill; maybe it would all go away.

That "magical thinking" didn't work. I *did* have cancer, and it was the radiation that made it "go away."

So, when I got prostate cancer, I no longer kept my illness a secret from friends and colleagues. And I felt better for it!

Some Tips for Coworkers of a Person with an Illness are:

○ Take your cues from the person who is sick. If he wants to talk about serious matters, then be a good listener. You can demonstrate your care and concern about what he is going through with a reassuring hug or even attentive silence. Try to anticipate needs so the person isn't placed in the awkward position of asking for even more help.

○ Understand that some drugs and treatments may have side effects, discuss such effects, and seek advice on how to respond.

—Bonnie Teitleman, director of the Faculty/Staff Assistance Program, and Nikki Sibley, director of the Office of Family Resources and Boston University Children's Center

IN A SENTENCE:

Whom you tell is up to you, but the more you talk about your illness and emotions, in general, the better you'll feel.

learning

Taking Charge of Your Health Care

ANY DECISION about your health care is the responsibility of you, the patient, and your family, though obviously in conjunction with your oncologist. This means that at all times you have the right to know as much about your case as you desire to, and that no treatment may be administered to you without your **informed consent**.

What does taking charge involve?

With prostate cancer, as you have undoubtedly gleaned by now, there are lots of unknowns, and lots of options. The multitude of factors may seem overwhelming at first, so here is how to organize your course of action.

- ○ Make sure that your doctors tell you everything they know about your case in particular and about available treatments and statistics/study results pertaining to it.
- ○ You also need to get your doctors to voice their opinion as to what you should do. Ask them _why_ they favor one treatment avenue over another. This should not offend

them. These days, with this kind of cancer, many urologists and oncologists very much want to leave the decision making to you, though they may be eager to pursue their own first choice.

○ Discuss this decision with as many people as you can: with members of your family; with other men who have had prostate cancer—with or without treatment; with friends who are physicians but whose specialty may not be oncology.

○ You may want to read opinions of other doctors or of researchers in the field, on Web sites or in books or magazines. For instance, you may want to educate yourself further about the controversy surrounding PSA tests.

○ You need to reconcile your present anxiety with feelings you might have tomorrow or the next day if you take one step or another. It's hard to wait for test results to kick in, but waiting can be important. It's not necessarily the same as doing nothing. You need all the information you can get about what is going on in your body. And moving ahead instead of delaying recommended treatment, once all that information is in, is just as important. Don't let "what ifs" paralyze you from coming to an informed decision.

○ You may want to start thinking about finding a support group, if you haven't done so before. There, you may find men who have made decisions about treatment, and have gone through that treatment. They can certainly give you important input into treatment options.

○ Finally, you need to remain calm and look very closely at the statistics I give in Month Six, so that you have as much real-world information as you can.

What I didn't do

It's necessary that I pause here to tell readers that I did *not* do as I'm advising you to do. I took my oncologist's recommendation and went ahead and had external beam radiation therapy. The result was a certain amount of comfort that I had "beaten" the cancer, but a certain amount of discomfort because of side effects. In addition, now that I've done all this research on watchful waiting, I think I might have chosen that three years ago, if I'd been more patient and waited to make up my mind.

Making the system work for you, not you work for the system.

Let's assume that you have gotten all the information that you can from doctors, friends, relatives, Web sites—not to mention this book. How do you take charge of your illness?

Half the battle here is deciding what kind of care—in the broader sense, not just the treatment per se—you want. Hearing out those closest to you, finding the right hospital and physician, learning about other prostate cancer patients' experiences—all that information is material you need to digest.

Among other things, you and your wife or partner should sit down and have a long discussion about all that is known and all that is unknown. You may want to select just one person—a physician who has had a profound influence on your life, a friend, a teacher, a psychotherapist—to help guide your decision making.

It's not easy, as I said. Your shock at hearing you have a malignancy may outweigh your normal coping tools. That's where friends and loved ones come in. My wife, the social worker, is fond of saying that when crises come, someone else often has to step in as the "ego" of the patient. For many men this is a terrible thought: we like to be autonomous, macho, strong, and in the catbird seat. But this may be one time where throwing the ball to someone else will actually allow you to make better decisions.

Working together, you and your wife/partner can get around some of the impediments to the best care. For example, if you want to see a doctor who's too busy, if you want to use a hospital that's not nearby, or if you want to circumvent the rules of your insurer's health plan—it may take joint efforts to do that. You may need to "work the system," which may be for you a whole other education in itself.

There are street-savvy techniques that may come in handy.

Like, don't take no for an answer.

Like, calling someone in a position of power (a congressman, a senator).

Like, finding out who is on the board of a hospital; you or someone you know may know them. (The minute I learned I had lymphoma years ago, I asked someone who knew the president of Memorial Hospital to phone and get me an appointment. I didn't want any problems or delays!)

You are your best patient's rights advocate, so don't be afraid to speak up.

Start with what you know

You already know a good deal about finding help for yourself. Over your lifetime, and that of your spouse or partner, you've looked for—and found—doctors who can take care of you. When looking for someone to help you get the best care now, and to help you get around obstacles to that care, go back and talk with your primary care physician. He may know little or nothing about prostate cancer (which is why you went to a specialist for your biopsy), but your personal physician knows you and what you want, and has colleagues in the field and at lots of medical institutions. Your hometown may not be the place to get your cancer treatment, but that doesn't mean that your hometown doctor doesn't have friends in high places elsewhere.

And those friends have colleagues and friends who might have valuable input or contacts. When you tap into this health-care network, you may just find a host of associates and specialists who could deliver the highest quality care for you. And they may squeeze you in because of a long-ago friendship with your hometown doc.

This is a good time to remember to slow down

It can be frustrating and anxiety producing to work your way through these systems, but keep in mind that your cancer took a long time to get to this size. It's going to take a long time to get much bigger. You can afford to get the right kind of care, the right people to talk with and by whom to be treated.

One doctor pointed out that if you gave yourself the power and the choices and the research with physicians in time of emergency that you do when buying a major kitchen appliance, you'd be in fine shape!

Don't leave everything to your doctor, with the excuse that you aren't a doctor. You can use all the skills you've developed over the years in your own profession to accomplish those goals. When we're sick, especially with "the big C," we sometimes begin to act like children; to turn responsibility over to others. We forget all our street smarts, our well-honed abilities that have served us in other spheres of life. Use them. They can get you far in this foreign land of medicine and health care.

The Dartmouth Atlas

The Dartmouth Atlas, about ten years in the making and still ongoing, began in Hanover, New Hampshire. Researchers who were trying to help patients make decisions in partnership with their physicians discovered an interesting fact: physicians in different localities proposed different treatments for the same illnesses. In other words, the kind of treatment most offered and most given for some illnesses varies greatly in different localities. This was true even when recent research showed some of these treatments not to be the most effective for those diseases.

For instance, *U.S. News* reports, "In California elderly Medicare enrollees in Palm Springs had double the rate of knee replacement surgery in 1999 than comparable Medicare patients did in Stockton." This reflects a wide variety of factors, many of which need not bother you. But the fact that different localities use different treatments for your cancer at your stage and your age should interest you. You may want to use the atlas to see where your community facilities stand. See the sidebar for details.

> **USE THE** Internet to go to the Dartmouth Atlas home page (www .DartmouthAtlas.org) and click "Search." Enter "prostate cancer" and look at the article that is likely to be the first one that comes up, called "Early Stage Prostate Cancer." That will lay out the demographics.

Remember, it's your decision, not your doctor's

At your age, and given your present anxiety, it may be difficult to argue with a man or woman who has a medical degree. But it is your body, your life, and your cancer.

If you don't think what you're being told reflects the alternatives or the thinking you've read about here—or on the Internet, or anywhere else—for God's sake, tell your doctor.

You don't have to be aggressive about this. You can, once again, use the skills you've honed when communicating with business associates or friends. Ask questions about other ideas and other treatments. These days, physicians are used to this.

And if you can't push past an obdurate system, get help in doing it. You may need to change doctors if yours proves unwilling to be upfront or open to other points of view, but think of it this way: would you rather you found that out about him now, when you have time and flexibility about your choices (even if he may not think so) or in a moment of true crisis?

Some way, somehow, you'll obtain the health care you need.

Staying in charge

In 2004, a book of mine was published that you may find helpful in this regard. Called *Staying in Charge* (John Wiley, 2004) it looks, among other things, at what ability and knowledge is needed where chronic illnesses are concerned.

Among the recommendations we make in that book is to find a health-care "agent." In the Learning section of Month Five, I'll deal with that in some detail. For now, however, my suggestion is that for those moments when perhaps you can't make decisions yourself, when you can't be in charge of your own illness—through fear, anger, despair, or just plain boredom from going through the ropes, not any major incapacity—find yourself someone who is willing and able to help you do research or objectively weigh your options. Someone who has "been there," who has traveled these roads before.

This can be a wife, a partner, a friend who is a nurse or administrator of a health-care institution—someone with stamina and knowledge. It's amazing how much help those who care about us can provide if we only ask.

IN A SENTENCE:

This is your disease; how to deal with it should be your decision.

WEEK **4**

Prostate Cancer and Sex

ERECTILE DYSFUNCTION (ED) is the term used by physicians. It's the term you'll hear over and over on television when they're selling you Viagra or Cialis. Perhaps the most famous person with ED is former senator and 1996 Republican presidential candidate Bob Dole, who made a commercial for Viagra.

I think the use of this term is a way of avoiding the painful word "impotence," but that it's important to keep things at the emotional level, for you to really feel them. "Impotence" is a more descriptive word—descriptive of the fact, and descriptive of the feelings associated with it. So, I'm going to use this word, not the euphemism ED, from here on.

Facing up to the possibility

The figures on who will or will not become impotent are confusing at best. To make a decision on treatment solely on the basis of whether you will or will not become impotent, you still would have to factor in your age, your general health, and the current statistics on likelihood of impotence from one procedure versus another. I was told there was a 35 percent chance of impotence with radiation, a 50 percent chance of it with surgery, and with "seeds" it was an unknown because they didn't have enough long-term studies. But, I was also told that it depended at which facility radiation was performed, and who did the seed implants. The reason is that some hospitals have more sophisticated equipment that can draw a 3D map of your abdomen and pelvis and place the seeds and/or shoot the radiation rays exactly where they're needed, avoiding other organs, while other hospitals aren't quite that sophisticated yet.

But even in the best of hands, stray bullets can happen, and slips can be made. And your anatomy is not as perfectly shaped as you would like it to be.

Which is how Tom Z. made what was for him the "right" decision, to have radiation at a major cancer hospital—yet became impotent nonetheless. Here's his story:

> About four months after radiation, when my prostate had shrunk, my PSA had dropped to 1.2, and my life was getting back to normal, I began to think again about having sex. I hadn't done it up to now because I discovered a certain amount of pain on the underside of my penis, near the tip, when I had an orgasm, and this made me somewhat leery of venturing out. To my dismay, when I now felt I wanted to, I could no longer get an erection.

For most of us the inability to have an erection when we want one is a devastating notion. It is not necessarily that we are sex addicts, nor that we need to have an orgasm. It is much more a symbolic event. Men have always associated their masculinity at least in part with their ability to have an erection and an orgasm.

Women say that the loss of a breast or the loss of ovaries deal a similar emotional blow. "I'm no longer a woman." "I can no longer have/nurse babies." Even women beyond the age of childbearing feel this burden.

You may be certain that, even if your wife or lover says your "erectile dysfunction" (as she will probably cautiously call it, if even that) doesn't bother her, it will bother *you*. Such impotence will make you feel, well, impotent. Powerless. Even though ED is discussed openly in TV commercials, the reality is that such shame is associated with the condition that men don't necessarily want to admit that they have a problem, physically or emotionally.

Impotence can be a devastating blow to men at any age that it occurs.

Whatever the myth, the truth is that sex is not just for people under thirty. If you're sixty-five or older, you'll know that the desire for sexual activity doesn't die with aging. It may mellow, or occur less often, but—from Kinsey forward—researchers have discovered what the aging population has always known: sex is part of our life.

Or at least we want it to be. If you've kept your interest in sex a tidy little secret, fine. That's between you and whomever you wish to share it with. But what is a pleasant secret when you're able to have erections, becomes an unpleasant secret when you're not.

And so you need to face that, despite the best efforts of your health-care team, you may experience some impotence after treatment for prostate cancer.

What is impotence?

In its most simple form, impotence is the inability to get an erection. It's important to understand that this definition of impotence refers to a whole series of medical malfunctions that can—and do—occur in men, without necessarily having to do with prostate cancer.

Let's begin by looking at the way erections occur.

You may remember from your high school or college biology class that there are two nervous systems—the **sympathetic** and the **parasympathetic**. It is the parasympathetic that causes **dilation** of arteries in a man's penis when he is sexually aroused. This arousal can come about by thoughts of sex as well as by actual physical contact by yourself or someone else.

For a variety of reasons, the veins in the penis act in concert with the arteries and cause an increase of blood pressure within the penis, which makes it engorge and enlarge.

When we are sexually stimulated, erections often occur without any thought or will on our part, that is, until some dysfunction occurs, at which time even the most persistent sexual touching or fantasizing may not create the swelling in our penises that comes with the other good feelings of sexual arousal.

Sometimes, a man will feel a warmth in his groin and the general feelings of arousal throughout his body, and then will be discouraged by realizing that his penis is not responding totally, or even at all. That is impotence.

Causes of impotence

It's important to learn that while some psychological problems can lead to partial or total impotence, it is much more often physical problems that are responsible. Merely knowing this often eases conflicts between husband and wife and relieves a sense of guilt or shame on the part of men. These causes may include:

○ Diabetes. It turns out that a high percentage of men with diabetes become partially or totally impotent.
○ Any problem of the circulatory system—and that includes the heart—can do the same.
○ Diseases of certain organs—such as liver and kidney can also contribute to impotence.
○ Parkinson's disease
○ Injuries to the back or pelvis
○ If you're a heavy drinker, or use drugs, or are grossly overweight, or a heavy smoker—all these can be contributors to impotence.
○ Then there are the medicines that have been prescribed for other problems you have, and about which you may not have been cautioned relative to their relationship to impotence. Believe it or not, this includes many of the over-the-counter and prescription medications to stop allergies; medications used for heart or circulatory problems; and drugs used to control mood disorders, such as anxiety or depression.

Impotence after treatment for prostate cancer

If you've been partially or totally impotent before treatment for your prostate cancer, you may already have talked with physicians or specialists about impotence. You may already be taking one of the fairly new medications to help relieve that condition.

None of that has to do, however, with the impotence that may occur after treatment, and it's about that I will now write.

All of the treatments we've talked about in Days Six and Seven, and Week Two, can cause impotence.

Surgery can damage the nerves and also the arteries that cause blood to flow more freely in your penis. Radiation can do the same. And hormones can change your nervous system's balance, to diminish the positive effect of your normal sexual arousal.

Impotence does not always occur right away, and one of the unfortunate things about the rhythm of treatment for prostate cancer is that you may have fully functioning erections for the first few months after surgery or radiation. Then, because scar tissue develops, or for many other medical reasons, the changes associated with diminished blood pressure or blood flow may set in. So, some men become impotent within three to four months after treatment has concluded.

This can be a shock, and without knowing such a delay is normal, some men or women will conclude that psychological problems are causing the impotence.

There is help

Your oncologist may be so used to hearing that a patient has become impotent after treatment that he may simply tell you to take Viagra and go no further. Conversely, a doctor may assume that it is not the treatment, but your depression over having the cancer that is at fault, and send you off to see a psychotherapist.

Both may be wrong; and both may be right.

That is why many men go elsewhere to find help for their impotence or—and this is sad—do nothing.

The result of doing nothing, of not asking for special help, is often a *real* depression about being "less" of a man, and this often hurts relationships between partners badly. We'll get to that issue in a bit. For now, let's deal with how you can go about treating this condition.

As with any medical problem these days, there are innumerable "answers" to your problem on the Internet. Dozens of Web sites will point you in the direction of this medication or that; or suggest additional surgery or mechanical devices. Let's look at some of those options; as with any treatment or procedure, be cautious about any claims that may sound too good to be true.

○ *Medicines on the market.* The three chief ones at this point are Viagra, Cialis, and Levitra. All three have the value of increasing blood pressure and flow to the penis, so that the normal arousal occasioned by sexual activity or thoughts can do its normal thing: enlarge and lengthen the penis. With each, there are pluses and minuses, some trumpeted loudly in advertisements, others not so loudly. In the fine print inside the container for each of these medications, you can get information about who is not supposed to take each medication, and what the side effects might be. At the moment, it's quite costly to take these pills, but many men will feel it's worth it if they have the desired effect.

○ **Pumps.** These devices can be purchased at "sex stores" or over the Internet. They vary widely in price—from $19.95 to $350—and vary in effectiveness as well, not necessarily related to price. The idea here is to create a vacuum in the penis, by drawing air into a pump that is fitted tightly over the penis. This pulls blood into the penis, causes an erection, and then a plastic ring is used at the base of the penis to retain blood in the penis long enough to have sexual intercourse or other sexual activity. I know this sounds like medieval torture, but men who have used pumps say that they can actually work if the impotence is not too severe. The expensive pumps may or may not work better than cheaper ones; may or may not be more comfortable; may or may not come with a guarantee. Deciding what to do is up to each user.

○ **Surgical inserts.** There are two kinds. The first is the insertion of a permanent rod into the penis. As you can imagine, this causes a permanent erection; the erect penis is held down by a restraint for normal life activities. The second is the insertion of a tiny air bag (for want of a better description) in the scrotum between the two testicles. When an erection is wanted, the man can inflate the bag, causing a self-contained fluid to flow into the penis. I have seen this in operation, and talked to someone who had one of these pumps. He declared it to be "miraculous" and said the doctor had "saved his life." For those for whom the idea of surgery on any part of their genito-urinary system is anathema, the insertion of anything into the penis or scrotum may be more than they want to think about. But the option is there. Medicare will pay for much of this cost, by the way.

How to choose a solution

There must be many thoughts going through your mind at this point, but the essential question I think you should focus on is, How do I make a choice between these options?

Be prepared for conflicting replies, even from your doctors. Bernard talked with his urologist, first, and received the stock answer: "Try Viagra. It may or may not help." He then went to his physician: "I can send you to a specialist in pumps." He saw the specialist, but this man was very dismissive of the hand pump and of Viagra. Bernard felt the doctor was trying too hard to sell him on the penile insert pump, requiring surgery, and backed away. "What about Cialis?" Bernard asked. "Well," said the specialist, "if Viagra hasn't worked and you don't get any kind of an erection normally, I doubt if anything will work except an insert. But here's a Cialis prescription. Try it and call me in a month." Bernard tried Cialis. To his delight and amazement, it provided a sufficiently large erection for him to regain sexual activity with his wife.

Doctors who haven't personally used these drugs or devices are only second-guessing how they may affect each individual, and of course a surgeon may have a certain leaning toward the benefits of surgery. Once again, as with all the choices you've had to make up until now, you need to talk to people who have had experience—in this case, with their own impotence. What—if any—solution have they chosen? How did they come to that decision? Did Viagra or another drug or alternative medication work? Partially? Completely? Did they consider using a pump or insertion? Did what they decided on satisfy their needs?

Be prepared that their answers may be encouraging or discouraging. Keep in mind that your own situation is entirely unique to your body and emotional makeup. For you, what to try and what will work depend entirely on your particular degree of impotence, and your particular degree of comfort with the options available. The point is, better to ask around than not ask and have to live with a problem that may be solvable.

Miracles do happen

There is one thing most doctors will not tell you, either because they don't hear about it from their patients, or because it isn't emphasized in the literature. I ran across it in my interviews with men, and found it on the NCI Web site:

Partial impotence can partially reverse itself without medication or pumps. I use "partial" twice because no one states that a *total* impotence (i.e., no change in the size of the penis at all) can reverse itself. And no one I know claims to have gone from partial impotence to total pretreatment erectile strength.

But there can be enough erection through sexual arousal to (a) allow for sexual intercourse; and (b) allow for other kinds of sexual pleasure. The stories I heard make it clear that men have been able to have a sufficient erection—despite posttreatment partial impotence—to make both themselves and their partners feel hope and pleasure again.

Still, any degree of impotence is difficult to take. The psychological effects of impotence can be enormous.

Nonphysiological causes

While the great preponderance of impotence is not caused by psychological problems, the fact is that some instances of impotence can be the result of one. This is highly individualized, but in general one can say that the impact of having radiation or surgery on your genitourinary system, the mere *suggestion* that you might become impotent, may in fact cause you to become impotent. If your physician suspects this may be the case, it's clearly worth your while to visit a psychotherapist.

For some people, grief counseling may be valuable to relieve the pain and anxiety associated with even *talking* about reduced sexual activity after prostate cancer treatment.

IN A SENTENCE:

> *Don't suffer in silence—discuss impotence with your partner, health-care team, and men who have experienced it.*

learning

Other Physical Side Effects

What kind of side effects might I expect?

I've touched on side effects before, but let's go over them again, all in one place.

The treatments I've talked about—surgery and radiation (beam or seed implantation)—can lead to some of the following:

O Diarrhea
O Cramping
O Fatigue
O Moderate bleeding
O Irritation of penis or rectum
O Impotence
O Incontinence
O Moderate pain

Not every patient, by any means, gets all of these side effects. And some patients actually escape most of them.

A survey of prostate cancer patients showed that, with prostatectomy, two-thirds had some urinary incontinence;

60 percent were "unable to have an erection firm enough for intercourse"; and 20 percent needed treatment caused by scar tissue in the urethra. These kinds of side effects are lessening as new surgical techniques are being brought into play.

With several exceptions, the symptoms are usually moderate, of short duration (a few weeks or months), and not a large problem. (Fatigue has already been discussed in Day Seven.)

Incontinence

Inability to hold urine, however, can be a major disruption in a person's life. The extent of incontinence following prostate cancer treatment varies greatly. Most men who receive seed implantation or carefully focused beam radiation do not become incontinent—but some do.

Many men who receive surgery do become incontinent, at least for a while. It's a matter of reduced muscle control, both in the urethra and in the bladder. Those muscles can become strong again after surgery, and control can be regained, thus for most men it is a temporary problem.

Briefly, there are three distinct kinds of incontinence. There is the kind that occurs from laughing, coughing, picking up heavy objects, etc. This causes a small amount of urine to escape because the **sphincters** that control the flow of urine from the urethra have been weakened.

If a man finds himself going to the bathroom often during the night, or not feeling "empty," it can be because the bladder muscles are weak, and the bladder becomes "too full." This can also happen without treatment for prostate cancer. Many men find this kind of incontinence is normal as they get into their seventies and eighties.

Perhaps the most unpleasant kind is "urge incontinence," which results in leaks that happen so quickly you can't get to the bathroom soon enough, or at night, and this can be embarrassing. This happens, too, with prostatic hyperplasia, but that can be corrected with surgery. Here, it is surgery that has weakened the bladder's muscles.

Countermeasures

There are several countermeasures that can be taken against incontinence:

- ◯ Exercises to strengthen muscles
- ◯ Medications to do the same
- ◯ Physical inserts to substitute for the malfunctioning sphincters

Your urologist can help you with all of these.

Where these three measures don't work, there are certainly other methods to handle your embarrassment, as well as the leakage of urine. As with impotence, it's crucial to learn how to adapt to incontinence, so that your life does not become constrained. Yes, it can be distressing to feel like you're out of control, but it's part and parcel of dealing with the entire mess of having prostate cancer.

Products

While I can list the products that are available, the most sensible thing to do is to go to the American Cancer Society Web site that deals with these matters: http://www.cancer.org/docroot/NWS/content/NWS_2_1x_Managing_Incontinence.asp, as well as their site called "Man to Man," which is a support group for men who have had treatment for prostate cancer. (Call 1–800-ACS 2345 for more information.)

The other side effects

For patients who are in pain, which can be a result of Stage III or Stage IV prostate cancer, see Month Seven's Learning section on pain control.

But there may also be times when irritation of parts of the genitals and rectum occurs because of a treatment for Stage I or Stage II prostate cancer, and here I want to give a few hints for dealing with them derived from the field of palliative care and the NCI. These can also be helpful for psychological irritation and pain.

- ◯ Professional massage. Everyone knows what massage is, but very few men go for massage therapy during happier times. As someone who learned about the pleasure of massage for aching muscles, tendinitis, and tired minds a long time ago, I can tell you that massage is doubly a relief when too much stress in your life is causing emotional or physical muscle pain. Finding a licensed massage therapist is simple. The Yellow Pages can direct you there. So can a local chiro-practor or physical therapist.

○ Home massage. As long as you're careful not to irritate skin already irritated by radiation or other procedures, the use of a vibrator at home can be almost as relaxing as a massage with a professional. Almost, but not quite.

○ **TENS machine**. The TENS device is inexpensive, handheld, and battery-operated. It delivers tiny beams of electricity to muscles that are frozen or knotted up.

○ Heating pad. An old remedy, but it works.

○ Cold packs. I assume you know that cold works best when muscles have just been injured; heat after the cold pack has reduced the knot. Try both.

○ **Acupuncture**. The tiny needles frighten away lots of men, but this ancient Chinese practice has been shown to alleviate many ail-ments, and it certainly works for pain. It has some of the same effects as a TENS machine but, in the hands of a skilled practitioner, can do wonders. One of the things I don't like about acupuncture, how-ever, is that its practitioners usually also prescribe and sell Chinese herbal remedies to you as an adjunct. Be aware that even herbal drugs are drugs; discuss such substances with your physician before taking them. Depending on what these are, they could be con-traindicated during and after treatments for prostate cancer, so cau-tion is imperative. Acupuncture should be beneficial without these adjunct medicines.

IN A SENTENCE:

Side effects are usually treatable and/or may recede with time.

FIRST-MONTH MILESTONE

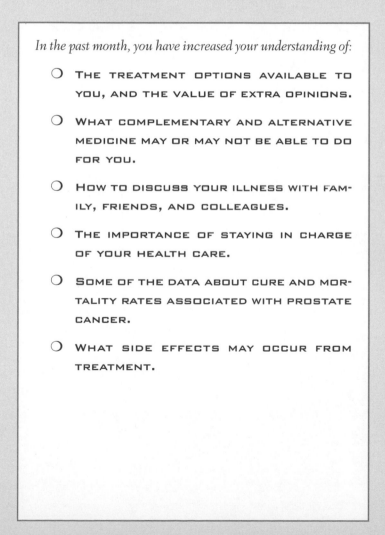

In the past month, you have increased your understanding of:

○ The treatment options available to you, and the value of extra opinions.

○ What complementary and alternative medicine may or may not be able to do for you.

○ How to discuss your illness with family, friends, and colleagues.

○ The importance of staying in charge of your health care.

○ Some of the data about cure and mortality rates associated with prostate cancer.

○ What side effects may occur from treatment.

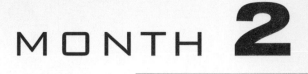
Dealing with Your Emotions

IN THE days and weeks before treatment begins, most men will feel some anxiety about a number of things: whether they've chosen the right treatment; how the treatment will go; whether they'll have any of those unpleasant side effects you've just been warned about.

You may not feel this emotion as anxiety. You might find yourself suddenly blowing up at your wife or kids. You may find yourself sleeping badly or, conversely, oversleeping. You may have an upset stomach. Or, if you're particularly sensitive, you may feel the anxiety more directly, as a tingling in your spine, a frazzled brain, a fried ability to perform normal duties. You may be able to express that anxiety directly to people around you. Or, you may not.

Jordan and Elizabeth were two weeks away from a course of radiation for his prostate cancer. "I'm fine," Jordan said. "You're not," answered his wife. He had gone to work as usual every day, and she was sure he was "braving it" just because he was a "macho man." Underneath, however, she saw a man who was worried sick about what was happening to him. Periodically, she tried discussing the matter with him, but he always protested that what he was feeling was "normal," and that it would go away as soon as he was treated.

Does this anxiety just go away?

The commencement of treatment sometimes alleviates anxiety. Sometimes not.

And what if it does? Why should you have to put up with it for the period that you're experiencing it—that is, if you even are willing to admit that you're anxious?

Jordan said, "Hey, you get frightened at heights. That's reasonable. There's nothing you have to do about that. And I don't need to do anything about this. It's normal. Who wouldn't be frightened about surgery?"

This is not an unusual response from men (or women) who are used to "toughing it out."

But let's ask if it really is necessary to put yourself through this. Do you have to experience these tough feelings just because what you're about to go through is what a lot of other people go through? And are you really experiencing just normal anxiety? Deep down, where it really counts, are you perhaps worrying about some things that you don't even need to worry about? Like death, for instance. Or impotence. Or incontinence. Those are things I don't like to think about. Such unreleased stress cannot only upset us emotionally and mentally, but can actually affect our body's health. There's more to this issue than most of us know about. A recent article in the *New York Times* discussed research that shows the mechanisms by which stress actually can cause our hair to turn white and age our bodies.[1] Also, it is now definitive that stress can cause disease in our bodies. And to add injury to insult, for men under seventy, researchers recently found that anger can cause strokes.

A form of counseling called cognitive therapy, in which people learn to temper their responses to stress, could help, psychologists say.

Beyond that, some patients actually begin to think of suicide at this point, or become paranoid. I've heard of men who cannot face the idea that their sex lives might be affected by their cancer. Others may begin to believe that the doctors are lying to them (either that they don't have cancer—and the hospital just wants to make money—or their cancer is much worse than the doctors are saying). These are radical reactions, ones you likely don't have, but they indicate the kind of emotional roller-coaster that can occur when you have been told you have cancer.

Jordan said to his wife, "What can a psychologist do? Nothing she'll say will take away the fact that I've got cancer and that I have to have treatment. Right?"

If you don't feel like your old self, or someone close to you indicates he or she is worried about your behavior, don't be too proud or stubborn to go for help. Get some counseling now. No, it won't cure your cancer—but it will help you live better with the fact that, for now, you have cancer.

For those of you who don't see the wisdom of getting some counseling or therapy, let me lay out what a therapist can do:

- She can help you determine just what your fears are—which ones are on the surface, and which are buried beneath the surface.
- She can help you examine whether these fears are justified.
- Assuming that they are justified, she can help you live with these fears by giving you her full attention. This supportive therapy can be surprisingly and wonderfully helpful.

Let's listen again to Charles:

During the time that I thought I'd have to pay for my treatment out of my pocket, or at the least a huge portion of it, I was very unhappy. I began to think my cancer was going to be worse than it actually was. I used to break into anger when my wife asked me for something, no matter how reasonable it was. I imagined going bankrupt. At the hospital, when I went for treatment, I used to blow up at very sweet medical assistants who didn't give me exactly what I needed.

So, I decided to get some help. I wanted someone who would understand what I was going through. I wanted someone who had seen men with prostate cancer. I found a woman and, surprisingly, I didn't find it difficult to talk to her at all. She had seen a number of men with prostate cancer. She knew the workings of hospitals.

What she did was not miraculous. She didn't get rid of my financial problem. She didn't get rid of my cancer. But just by telling me how many people go through this with the same kind of fears; by pointing out that everyone knew that my hospital was not helpful on financial matters; and by listening to my worries— I felt like a miracle had occurred.

I became less anxious, less angry. And, believe it or not, I became more effective in solving my own problems.

Charles needed only four or five sessions with his counselor to accomplish his goals. He was totally happy with what they did together.

What has been long established is that to the extent you can find someone to talk to about anxiety or other emotional problems that are not long-standing but are situational, not only will your present life be made more palatable, but your treatment outcome may be, too.

How's that for a win-win solution?

IN A SENTENCE:

Emotional upsets are common, but you don't have to live with them.

learning

Finding a Therapist

I **PERSONALLY** have had enough psychotherapy and counseling in my life to come to believe that it's easy to find the "right" person to talk to. Oh, yes, my wife happens to be a social worker who is a psychotherapist. That helps. But many people don't have that luck or that experience.

How do you find a therapist?

In much the same way that you went about getting the right hospital and getting a second opinion, you can find the right counselor or therapist for yourself. Let's start by talking about what kind of help you need.

There are several kinds of therapists and counselors. "Counselor," by the way, is a fairly nonspecific title. It refers to anyone to whom you might talk about a problem, be he or she a marital counselor, a priest, or a trained psychotherapist. "Therapist" refers to one of several kinds of people who have gotten a degree in psychological approaches to people's problems. The most common titles you will recognize are:

- Psychiatrist
- Psychoanalyst
- Social worker
- Psychologist

A psychiatrist is a person with a medical degree who has taken additional training in psychological problems, and holds a second degree in that work. A psychoanalyst is generally a psychiatrist who has taken "analytic training" for an extended period of time.

The social worker has a master's degree in social work from an accredited institution, usually with a variety of training, including psychotherapy. A psychologist has a PhD from a college and must also have training in psychotherapy. Neither of these latter kinds of counselor is an MD. Sometimes, with additional training, a psychologist can be what is called a "lay" analyst, i.e., a psychoanalyst who is not a physician.

While any one of these people may be able to help you with the impact of impotence upon your life, if what you're depressed about is clearly the aftermath of your treatment for prostate cancer—in other words, if you were a fairly well-adjusted man before the diagnosis—then I'm not suggesting here that you seek a psychoanalyst. That practitioner is usually interested in the deeper conflicts of people for whom there has been an early life trauma, or who have serious underlying problems that are long-term, and which need long-term treatment.

While either a psychologist or a social worker might be a successful counselor on this matter, the benefit of going to a psychiatrist is that he or she will have some of the underlying medical knowledge that can help you understand what is due to your treatment and what is not.

However, there are other good and sufficient reasons for choosing a psychologist or social worker.

One is the fact that many more people seek therapy from social workers than from any of the other practitioners in this country. Social workers are the front line of help in the mental health field and, consequently, see a large number of people, and thus have a great deal of experience in many arenas. Social workers cost less, and in these days of managed care, you might find it easier to find, to see, and to pay for a social worker than other specialists.

Julio happened to obtain his treatment at a hospital that had a number of social workers who were there specifically to deal with the psychological dilemmas of patients. He learned about this opportunity from the "patient representative" at the hospital. Many hospitals now have such a department: employees of the hospital whose job it is to listen to any kind of patient's problems—financial, personal, administrative—and try to solve them. In the course of discussing one of the administrative problems he faced, Julio asked if the rep could tell him where he might find a good counselor, and he was directed to Joyce S., a social worker at the hospital.

Within a day, he had an appointment with Joyce. To his delight he discovered that there was no cost for this service, because he was already a patient there. He also was pleased to find that she had dealt many, many times with patients who had prostate cancer.

IN A SENTENCE:

> *Several different kinds of counselors could help you manage your emotions.*

living

How to Pay for Treatment

IT IS likely that you will be able to afford the best treatment in at least one of four ways:

1. You are employed and have health insurance with a good company.
2. You don't have a lot of money, but you're on Medicaid.
3. You're not retired, not employed, but have your own individual or family insurance.
4. Or, you're over sixty-five and on Medicare. Preferably, with a "Medigap" insurance policy.

Even if you fit into one of those categories, it could still be a challenge to obtain the care you believe is best if, for instance, the specialist or hospital you have chosen is a thousand miles away and/or not in your health plan.

In such an instance, depending on your insurance plan, you are likely to get some reimbursement, but that "some" may be 80 percent of reasonable costs, where what is reasonable to your health plan is not what is reasonable to you; i.e., you will have to pick up the tab for any medical procedures your insurer deems unreasonable. And then there's the 20 percent copayment. If you will be getting surgery or radiation—those costs can mount into the tens of thousands.

So, while all of the above options should provide you with good coverage, there are always going to be glitches. And how you get around these glitches will depend on knowing about them ahead of time, as well as being dogged on your own behalf.

Let's start with the glitch that I discussed to some extent on Day Three, when I talked about your search for the best hospital and doctor. If you have an HMO, or another kind of managed care, you may have opted for a system that limits who may treat you and where you can obtain treatment. This is clearly a way for the managed care company to save money. But it can be a problem for you. Say, you've decided to go to a hospital in another city, or to a doctor who specializes in prostate cancer at a particular center that is not on your HMO's list.

What are your options at this point? One option is that you can choose to use the doctor and hospital that you want, and pay the out-of-network fees associated with that. You won't be reimbursed for the 80 percent of the bill that would be if you used an in-system doctor or hospital. You can fight your HMO on this, but whether you win or not will depend on several factors:

○ How good you are at fighting.
○ How determined the managed-care company is to hold the line.
○ Whether a court case has decided in their favor previously.
○ How much extra money we're talking about!

Here's another scenario:

You've opted for a new treatment, or one that the HMO thinks is not proven. Or, after a year, your physician says you need another diagnostic test and, for some reason, either Medicare or your HMO says, "we don't pay for those until *two* years have passed."

The first thing to do with this is to go immediately to your doctor or his administrative assistant. Tell them the story, and see if they can "code" the test or treatment differently. This is NOT, (repeat NOT) illegal or scandalous. There are many codes that reflect your particular needs and your diagnosis. Sometimes all that's needed is to make sure that your hospital or physician has thought carefully about how to code it. For example, did they put down the numbers that represent "colonoscopy because of previous cancer" or did they put down the code that just says "colonoscopy"?

Another possibility: Go directly to your HMO or to Medicare and protest.

In the worst-case scenario, listen to Charles, who had a problem that refused to get solved:

> The year I turned sixty-five, I went to my local social security office and signed up for Medicare. My birthday was in March, but, as suggested by the government, I signed up in December of the year before. I was asked whether I wanted to sign up for Part B—the optional part of Medicare for which you pay a fee, and that covers outpatient doctors' office or hospital costs. Either because I was stupid or because of a lack of understanding, I said "no." After receiving my card, someone at my office told me that I should have signed up for Part B. Since I was still within the sign-up period, I wrote a letter to Medicare, telling them to reverse my decision.
>
> Time passes. I turn sixty-five. March, I'm diagnosed with prostate cancer. Tests and radiation are scheduled and, to my horror, I'm told that I'm not covered for these expensive procedures *because I don't have Part B of Medicare.*
>
> I went to the hospital administrator, thinking that he would help me sort this out. He was less than helpful. His interest was in getting paid, and the hospital would, in fact, get paid MORE if I paid out of my pocket than if Medicare paid.

Here's how that works. Major medical centers make a deal with Medicare: they will accept so many dollars for this procedure and so many for that. It's not their choice; it's Medicare's. If your hospital wants Medicare patients, they have to agree that this is what they'll accept for each operation or other procedure. This is generally much lower than an individual would pay if he or she had no insurance, and a different figure even than what a managed care company will pay. At least in the case of the HMO, the deal is struck between hospital and insurance company. In the case of Medicare, it's a take-it-or-leave-it negotiation. So, while I can't promise you that this executive was actually thinking about the money the hospital would make if Charles paid out of his own pocket, (as opposed to Medicare,) the fact is there was no incentive for him to help Charles—except to be a nice guy in his time of need.

> I can tell you my anxiety level went through the roof! Finally, I contacted one of my senators. A wonderful woman in his office handled the matter immediately, and within a week I had a letter from Medicare saying I was covered for Part B from March, in other words, from before any of my treatments for cancer. What a relief!

It wasn't that Charles did anything wrong, though he felt guilty toward his family, and furious at himself for having declined Part B in the first place. Rather, the lesson here is that mistakes happen, and the system isn't very forgiving. The system is also not very helpful if it doesn't want to be. Let me correct that statement: The system isn't very helpful if certain people in charge don't want it to be.

That brings us back to the four options I described at the beginning of this chapter, and one of the problems with the American health-care system: What if you have a little bit of money, but not enough to be on Medicaid?

Medicaid rules

How Medicaid works is beginning to change. The second round of cuts in federal budgets in 2005 is making states rethink how much they can afford to pay people for medical costs they can't afford. But one thing is not likely to change: the rule about what it means not to have enough.

Some years ago, people were finding they could sign their money and assets away to family members one day and apply for Medicaid the next. The government plugged that loophole. A law made it pretty much the rule universally throughout the United States that you have to have given away your assets (with a few exceptions, like your house) and be living on a fixed income (or with stipends from a trust held by your family) for three years before you apply for Medicaid support. This rule makes it unlikely that a person can discover he has prostate cancer in March, and apply for Medicaid funds in May.

This means that if you have some funds and assets, but paying for your treatment would bankrupt you or give you extreme financial duress, yet you don't qualify for Medicaid (there are limits on how much money you can have), you face a terrible dilemma.

What many people have had to do at that point is to sell their house, move in with family, or forgo the treatment they need. Another option here is to join a clinical trial. I'll get to that in detail in the Learning section of this chapter.

Not all insurance policies are alike

If you have never sat down and read through not only your health insurance policy but the other plans your insurer offers, this is the time to do it. Most insurers issue an array of plans, with different levels of deductibles, copayments, and levels of care. The one with the least monthly fee may not include prescription drugs or other features that a higher grade will cover. Generally, you are allowed to change from one level to another at a fixed time once per year, when the policy is renewed. If such a change might result in greater coverage for a treatment plan you are considering, it might be worth waiting a month or two to be able to switch insurance plans.

One caveat: Whatever plan you have signed up for, you may want to hold off any test that can identify whether you carry the gene that demonstrates susceptibility for prostate cancer, unless you are absolutely sure taking the test will not become grounds for your insurance carrier to cancel your policy, which can be the case if women test positive for the BRCA1 gene. Don't jeopardize valuable coverage without checking first whether the company takes that stance.

What if you're still working

I want to talk briefly about what happens if you still have a job and are covered under your employer's insurance plan. This can occur even if you're over sixty-five and your employer has a certain number of employees. Your Part A (inpatient hospital) coverage is automatic once you start getting social security payments. Your Part B is not, and it's under outpatient coverage that you would be reimbursed for radiation, hormone therapy, and many other cancer treatments.

It would be best if this discussion had come up some years or months back, when you could check with your personnel office without having treatment already looming over your shoulder. But now is better than after treatment. Find out from your human resources officer what your coverage would be for each of your treatment options. That way, you won't go into treatment blind, without knowing what your reimbursement will be.

IN A SENTENCE:

> You need to read your insurance and other health-care policies carefully to assess what will and will not be covered.

learning

Is Joining a Trial Study for You?

What is a clinical trial?

Before the use of any new treatment and before medication is allowed to be prescribed, it has to be put to a variety of tests. Traditionally, with drugs for instance, this includes what's called a **double-blind study**. Used for decades in the field of medicine and psychology, such a study creates two (or more) randomly assigned groups of subjects or patients. One group is given the new treatment. Another is given a **placebo**. Yet another may be given another substance for comparison.

None of the groups knows which treatment it's getting. After studying the effects upon each group, a statistical analysis will determine whether the new drug is as effective, more effective, or less effective than the placebo or another medication.

Effectiveness is a crucial quality, but it is not the only one. Testing for safety is also important, and most studies want a long enough period after using the drug to see what negative side effects might develop. The same is true of studies for new treatment techniques.

With cancer treatments, however, since a person's life is at stake, it is hard or impossible to find anyone who would want to participate in a study where a placebo is used.

Consequently, for ethical and humanitarian reasons, the new treatment is compared with a treatment already in use. And in such cases, the participants know which they're getting.

This kind of study is called a clinical trial. These trials are usually conducted under the auspices of major organizations—and very often financed by the federal government, rather than by private industry, though occasionally, when a **proprietary** technique or piece of equipment is involved, that might occur.

The benefits of clinical trials

To the uninitiated, the idea of being a "guinea pig" in a clinical trial often sounds absurd: "Why should I try something unproven, when there are many good treatments around that work?" one man asked.

The answer comes in several parts, though perhaps the word "work" should be looked at first. What "work" means can be viewed through different prisms, depending on your point of view. It can mean, "gets rid of all the cancer." It could mean, "It keeps me from dying." It could mean, "It gets me through the next five years." For now, let's simply say that "work" means, "It's been tried before, it's safe, and it does seem to get rid of some or all of the cancer." With that definition in mind, why might you wish to participate in a clinical trial?

○ Since no treatment for prostate cancer is without some risk of side effects, researchers are always looking for safer and easier and less expensive ways of doing things. You might find a clinical trial with a new treatment that fits that bill.

○ The clinical trial is free. All treatments, tests, and drugs will be given to you. This can mean a life-saving situation for some men who may not have sufficient insurance to pay for expensive current treatments.

○ Some forms of prostate cancer—more advanced ones—do not respond to known treatments. Your physicians may suggest a clinical trial in which a promising new treatment for advanced prostate cancer is being tried out.

○ Clinical trials take place under very rigorous conditions. The protocols are carefully followed. You will have many researchers, nurses, and doctors looking out for your well-being, and you can generally be assured that the treatments will be carried out with the utmost care and diligence.

○ Often, clinical trials are carried out by the top researchers in the field. If you can be the recipient of a brand-new treatment that works, why not do it?

○ Finally, you will be told everything you can possibly want to know about what researchers already have found out about the risks, advantages, side effects, and other aspects of the treatment you're signing up for. And you will have plenty of opportunity to discuss these with your own oncologist, and to sign—or decline to sign—an informed consent form.

Reasons to avoid a clinical trial

○ If you or your doctor have doubts as to the value of the trial.

○ If you and your doctor feel that current, proven treatments will do enough for you.

○ If your cancer is "run of the mill" prostate cancer, and can be treated without risk with current treatments.

○ If you have any anxiety about being in a trial.

○ If you ask questions about the protocol, and don't feel you're getting the kinds of answers you require from nurses or doctors associated with the trial.

○ Finally, you may not be eligible for a particular trial because you don't fit the pattern of men they're looking for. This can be true especially if your cancer isn't of the type they think the new treatment will help.

Where can you learn more about clinical trials?

Browsing the Internet one day, I found an interesting Web site, CancerTrialshelp.org. (The .org designates a nonprofit organization. When it comes to getting help on the web, it's generally true that you'll get more authentic information from a .org than from a .com.)

I can't vouch for CancerTrialshelp.org, but I can say they have a lot of interesting material, so here's some of what you might do on that site:

○ They have a "User's Guide" link that includes the National Cancer Institute's list of ongoing cancer clinical trials.

○ Check their section called "Participating in a Trial: Questions to Ask Your Doctor."

○ They give all sorts of other details about clinical trials, including the fact that you can change your mind and leave the study whenever you want—before the study starts or at any time during the study or follow-up period. The NCI keeps an up-to-date list of all trials that are ongoing or coming up.

In the area of prostate cancer, we're told that as many as twenty new procedures are being tested or are going to be tested, and I found over 106 ongoing studies. The NCI tells us that the following clinical trials have been studied and are continuing to be studied for efficacy, safety, and long-term value, but they are by no means the only ones. Many combinations of chemical and biological agents are being tried with various stages of cancer.

Cryosurgery

Cryosurgery freezes cancer cells in the prostate. This sounds painful, but steps are taken to make sure you don't feel the liquid nitrogen that is used. You would stay in the hospital for a couple of days for this procedure.

Long-term results are not yet clear, though one certain side effect is impotence. It has occurred in nearly 100 percent of tests done so far. So you might want to keep away from this kind of clinical trial, at least until subsequent tests demonstrate that the side effect is eventually reversible.

Hormones

Hormone therapy is a useful treatment for metastatic prostate cancer, since it slows the disease down; though hormones won't cure it.

Clinical trials of the use of hormones in less radical or serious cancer are now taking place.

The idea is to slow the growth of the malignant cells so they don't spread more quickly into lymph nodes or other tissue or organs. Sometimes hormones will be given before surgery, in the same way that radiation is given after surgery. The hormones will shrink the tumor, so less has to be taken out by the surgeon.

A well-known case of this kind of treatment is former New York City mayor Rudolph Giuliani.

Ultrasound

It was previously believed that ultrasound was not useful in the treatment of cancer, but a new technique, called High Intensity Focused Ultrasound (HIFU), is being tested under FDA guidelines in the United States. For its acceptance in Europe, see Month Eleven.

Chemotherapy

According to the NCI, "Several promising new anticancer drugs are under study, being added to either surgery or radiation therapy for men with Stage III prostate cancer. Chemotherapy is also being tried in conjunction with hormonal therapy for men whose advanced cancers are no longer responsive to hormonal therapy alone."

Antiangiogenic therapy

This fascinating clinical trial is looking at the process of blood vessel formation. When new vessels are permitted to develop, cancer cells multiply and spread. The idea of antiangiogenic inhibition is the use of chemicals to prevent the blood vessels from being created. The theory is that doing so may make tumors shrink or disappear.

Complementary therapies

Another interesting Web site is psa-rising.com, which is billed as a "news, information and support" site for prostate cancer "survivors."

Like all Internet sites, caution should be taken when using the information found there, but a news report as impressive as the following should not be dismissed out of hand:

A new study at Northwestern University seeks to determine whether natural tomato oil with a high concentration of lycopene may reverse or delay progression of high-grade prostatic intraepithelial neoplasia, a condition in which abnormal cells form within the prostate and which is the strongest risk factor yet identified for the development of prostate cancer.[1]

Preliminary research has shown an over 20 percent reduced risk for developing prostate cancer in men who ate more cooked tomato products, such as tomato sauce. The National Cancer Institute–sponsored study at Northwestern will use tomato extract (literally, tomato oil) from non–genetically modified tomatoes raised in Israel and specially grown to be high in lycopene content.

According to one of the researchers at Northwestern, "Prostate cancer is a rational target for chemoprevention because of its high public health burden and relatively slow growth rate."

"Although early surgical treatment of prostate cancer might be effective, it involves substantial discomfort. This, plus the wide variability in the biological behavior of prostate cancer, makes overtreatment a persistent and serious concern," he added.[2]

Another study is looking at pomegranate juice, which may contain substances that decrease or slow the rise of PSA levels and may be effective in delaying or preventing recurrent prostate cancer.

Exercise caution: what you don't know can hurt you

While some prostate cancer patients feel that they benefit from some of these experimental therapies, before you try any of them, you should discuss their possible value and side effects with your medical doctors, particularly if you desire to test them while you are also receiving conventional treatments. You should definitely let them know if you are already dabbling in using any such therapies outside the controlled supervision of a clinical trial. Foods, herbals remedies, and so on, can interact with conventional medications in ways that could skew the benefits of either or both treatments.

Also, as with any treatment, you should ask the therapist sponsoring an ongoing trial for concrete evidence of how the therapy has helped others. Don't be misled by testimonials unsupported by at least preliminary hard data.

Be aware that these new therapies may be expensive, and some are not paid for by health insurance. On the other hand, if your insurance company is not providing the coverage you need for conventional treatment, entering a clinical trial could be doubly advantageous.

IN A SENTENCE:

> *Clinical trials are carefully run and offer many benefits beyond those of traditional treatments.*

MONTH 4

Keeping Up Your Strength

YOU'VE BEGUN treatment, or have taken a supervised wait-and-see attitude. What can you do to aid yourself physically?

If you already exercise at least three times a week for at least 20 or 30 minutes per session; if you eat a good deal of protein, and not too much fat; if you get a good night's sleep—well, you can just continue that process now.

If you aren't, what are you doing to keep otherwise healthy? Are you lying about, feeling bad and getting more and more tired? If you are experiencing any of the following—

○ You're having trouble sleeping.
○ You're tired during the day, and I mean *really* fatigued.
○ You aren't hungry.
○ You're eating a lot of junk food.
○ You aren't exercising at all.

—now's the time to admit as much to your doctor. Don't wait. Don't think, "Oh, what the hell, I've been through a lot, what's a gym or diet going to do for me now?"

Because what the researchers have found is that the more you let yourself go, the more you give up on what's recommended, the more likely it is that you'll continue to feel lousy tomorrow. Your doctor will probably recommend a mild physical regimen and also a diet plan, to strengthen your body against the cancer and to help your system hold up against the invasiveness of surgery, medications, or radiation.

The facts about exercise

You may already have a personal trainer, or go to a gym, or go out running three times a week, or play tennis, or any of those other activities that keep your heart working the way it's supposed to. But there's another, somewhat surprising fact that has come out recently about exercise.

In one study, it turned out that men who got exercise while having radiation for prostate cancer didn't feel as tired from the treatment as men who didn't. They were healthier all around, too.[1]

The problem is that once the fatigue from radiation gets going, it multiplies in effect. I didn't know this when I had my radiation, but because I kept going to work throughout my treatment, and kept working with my trainer, I know that I felt better throughout and afterward than were my friends who had the same treatment. Everyone said I was "brave" to keep working, but the fact was I felt better physically and mentally.

An independent researcher, when asked about the study, said that it turns out that exercise may also help men who are having hormone therapy because hormones can weaken bones and muscles.[2]

Cancer is a whole new ball game, and even whatever workouts you've done to keep in good shape in the past may need to be adjusted now. And if you've done nothing before, you really want to think about taking it up now.

Of course, you may not feel that you can exercise full out during your treatment. Don't be concerned. The study referred to above found that even a little bit of exercise makes a difference. It is vital to keep your muscles working. Lack of exercise weakens muscles, and that has a multiplying negative effect on your body.

The study's results do not mean that you have to become an exercise freak. You may be slim and trim without ever going to a gym. That's terrific. But then, you may not be.

One of the suggestions for men who aren't up to rigorous exercise—or who hate it—is the old Chinese practice of Qi Gong (pronounced "Chi Kong").

Qi Gong

The philosophy of this medical practice has to do with the power of breath to control physical well-being. Well, "breath" isn't quite right. It's the power of *qi,* a substance that supposedly circulates through the body and can make you well if it's nurtured. Tai Chi comes from this philosophy.

Understanding Qi Gong's ancient roots isn't necessary to gain benefits from it. And one of the best things about it is that it doesn't take a lot of time, and it isn't exhausting. That, for some of us, is a great thing.

Advocates say that it helps with strengthening muscles, allows for more oxygen to get into your lungs, and improves circulation. So, try it.

Here's a simple Qi Gong exercise:

Sit or stand upright. Keep your head a little higher than normal, but don't exaggerate it. Now, just swing your arms and hands from a downward vertical position to about halfway horizontal. In other words, they get only halfway up to your waist.

Let them fall back down. Continue this motion—up and down—at a pace equal to once every second or so (slower, if it's hard to keep up, but never faster).

Let everything be straight—your elbows, your fingers, your body.

It doesn't matter when you do this exercise, but make sure you're not cramming it into a small hole in your schedule. Part of the benefit here is mental, so you want to be able to take time away from your daily rush to do this.

After you've gotten it so that a five-minute Qi Gong session is fairly easy, increase to ten minutes. And so on, up to 30 minutes. If you can do this three times a week, you'll get tremendous benefits from it.

And if it hurts one day, or you feel exhausted, don't do it for the next day or so.

See how easy that was!

What if you feel really, really tired?

Take naps. I take one most days when I'm feeling tired—around 3 PM —but, then, I work from home, so it's easy for me to do. If you work at an office, see if there is a place where you can at least close the door for a while and rest sitting down (and by rest I mean do absolutely nothing but be sitting down—no phone, no computer). Or see whether you can shave some time off your workday—when it begins, when it ends—so that you can sleep longer at night.

When you know you're going to have to be active all day, you might be interested in a medication called Provigil (available only from a physician), a modern pick-me-up that's supposed to be safe and easy to use. My **psychopharmacologist** prescribed it to keep me going all day. It has no attendant jitters (like caffeine or amphetamines), and no adverse side effects, if taken early in the day.

But if, even with these kinds of measures, your fatigue is getting out of hand, or your wife, friends, or colleagues, people who know your usual personality well, are commenting on your withdrawal—something else could be going on. You may be depressed.

Why are you depressed? Because you've been through a very traumatic experience. It's no joke being told that you have cancer. No matter how strong you are, no matter how emotionally fit, even if you've had surgery, followed by radiation or preceded by hormones, or are under the latter treatments as a primary regimen, there may remain a doubt in your mind that everything's under control, that you are okay. You may not be aware of this doubt consciously (the human mind is great at hiding things like that), but it may be there nonetheless.

And if you've had only (!) radiation, which in of itself is a lot of treatment to take and can make you feel lousy, the downside of a treatment you cannot actually see or feel working is that it is way too easy to believe maybe it isn't working.

And let's not forget that the area that is being treated is one that is a man's very personal and important arena . . . I didn't want anyone fooling around with my reproductive system, thank you. How about you?

You may also be anticipating something else happening that you've read about. Like impotence. Or metastases. Or you may have some physical problems that were caused by the treatment, and it's hard to imagine now that they will lessen or go away.

Doctors and nurses try to follow up regularly. And when they do, they ask all sorts of questions about your health. But that doesn't mean they catch everything. And if you've got a little blood in your urine, or diarrhea, or you aren't sleeping well, that needs to be reported to your doctor. Don't assume everything will be fine just because you don't mention minor problems. You want to get on with the rest of your life, and if something is keeping you from doing that, it is not trivial or a sign of moral weakness. Get help.

IN A SENTENCE:

Don't neglect your overall physical health while attending to your cancer.

learning

Nutrition

AS YOU prepare for your treatment—making decisions about what kind to have, and anticipating a period of convalescence—you will begin to think about what you should eat during that time.

Let's begin with what is known about nutrition and prevention of cancer. Whatever I can tell you in that area would also stand you in good stead as you go forward. Since prostate cancer is a chronic, not a terminal, disease, you need to learn how to keep yourself healthy for many more years, not just for the present!

According to NCI booklets and Web sites, it is not at all clear that any major change in diet would have prevented your cancer. The caveat here, of course, is the assumption that you've been eating a balanced diet, with appropriate daily portions of fruits and vegetables high in antioxidants, and one that is low in animal fats. In addition, the assumption is that you aren't eating too much: one of the few nutritional facts that is known about prostate cancer for sure is that obese men are more likely to get the disease than men who are of "normal" weight.

What's a "balanced diet?"

Men are nowhere near as good about reading up on diets and food nutrition as are women, and may be bad eaters or overweight, without being aware of it.

So, perhaps it pays to give a few paragraphs over to a discussion of good eating and good nutrition in general.

Habits are hard to break, and food habits are some of the hardest, so nothing I'm going to say here will be radical in nature. You should be able to be a healthy eater without changing your diet in a major way. What I will do here is to point out what's good for you and what's not. It's up to you to do the rest. Just remember, when it comes to diseases, and to cancer especially, you want to eat so as to stay healthy, to avoid serious illness, and to stay strong during any treatment.

What is good for you

Vegetables and fruits are good for you. The darker the green in green foods, the more vitamins they have; in fact, as colorful a "palette" of produce as you can eat regularly, the better. Meat with low fat content, like chicken white meat, veal, and lean pork, are better for you than juicy (i.e., fatty) hamburgers. Turkey has less fat than chicken.

Fish is good for you. In fact, very good for you.[3]

Baking, roasting, and broiling (or grilling) is better for you than frying. I know that fried foods taste better, but the oil you fry them in is not healthy.

Eating food sprinkled with herbs and spices is better for you than lots of thick, rich sauces; however, tomato sauce or salsa are OK.

Low-fat cheeses, butters, and no-fat half-and-half do exist and are better for you than regular butter, cream, and lots of regular cheeses.

Don't eat sugar-heavy desserts. Do eat desserts made with sugar substitutes, or fresh fruit. Real fruit is better for you than juices, which again are loaded with sugar.

How you eat

Believe it or not, your mother was right: eating slowly actually helps you cut down on how much you eat, because your stomach takes a little while to react to the food that's coming down the pipe. If you eat your whole meal in ten minutes, your stomach may still say, "I'm hungry."

If you want a snack, try not to grab packaged snacks or cookies. Reach for carrots with low-calorie mayonnaise, for instance; or celery with peanut butter. Or fruit. Or a small amount of nuts, which are high-calorie but pack a lot of protein, and you need extra protein right now to help your body heal.

And grazing—that is, eating six or seven minimeals a day—is better for you than huge meals.

Drinking

My father drank a lot of alcohol. Toward the end of his life he weighed 220 pounds, didn't exercise, didn't eat much at meals, and died a miserable death.

Most soft drinks and all alcoholic beverages are bad for you.[4] Sorry. But that's the truth. Sugar-free (i.e., "diet") beverages are much better for you. And "light" beer is better than Guinness stout. But see if you can get into the habit of drinking just water sometimes: do you really need the sugar or alcoholic kick from a beverage, or are you merely thirsty? Still or carbonated water may well do the trick, to keep you hydrated without the calories.

Home cooking

One way to control your diet is to do more home cooking, from fresh ingredients (that is, not using prepared foods that you just zap in a microwave or heat in a pot), using some of the many gourmet cookbooks available for people who seek low-fat or low-carb meals. Not to knock restaurants, but it is far too easy while dining out to eat too great a portion, or to choose high-calorie, highly sauced, or otherwise unhealthy foods. If you stock your fridge and pantry with only . . . OK, mostly . . . healthy ingredients, you will eat well in spite of yourself. Eating out makes it easy to fall off the dietary wagon.

Are you overweight?

It doesn't take much self-perusal to discover if you're overweight or not. If you're about six feet tall, and you weigh anywhere from 140 to 180 pounds, you're in the normal range. Getting up over 200 pounds, you'd have to be six foot six for that to be healthy. It's that simple.

Well, what if you don't exercise and you're overweight? And you can't control your eating habits, because they've been going on too long. And you're not worried about this "little" bit of prostate cancer you have? You need to be worried. Every shrug of neglect is counteracting your treatment's working optimally against the malignancy. Call for help. See a nutritionist, or seek out one of the diet specialists your doctor might recommend. Or see a psychotherapist or social worker. Get your weight under control and you and your loved ones will be happier and healthier.

Can cancer be prevented through nutrition?

There are some ideas floating around about nutrition and dietary supplements, about which you will want to make your own inquiries. In fact, it might not be a bad idea to get your doctor to recommend a dietitian: someone who really knows the ins and outs of what your body might need in this particular circumstance.

Lycopene and tomatoes

Of all the natural foods, the one that may have a preventive effect on prostate cancer is the fruit we call a vegetable: the tomato. It contains a substance called lycopene, an antioxidant, which a number of studies and some anecdotal evidence show might be effective in preventing or slowing the progress of prostate cancer.

The facts are not all in by any means, and studies and trials are presently in motion to determine scientifically if this is so, but since tomatoes in any form are a very healthy thing to eat, there is no harm in increasing your intake of these, should you wish to, particularly in cooked form, which seems to better release the lycopene. Like anything that you do, however, moderation is the key word.

Selenium

This is a mineral that can be found in meats and other animal products. It helps antioxidant **enzymes** do their job. If you don't have enough selenium, you may get muscle pain. If you have too much, you can lose hair, or have skin problems. What's important in relation to this book, however, is that some evidence has come forward to suggest that selenium supplements can prevent some prostate cancers and slow down others.

The evidence from a number of studies suggests that if it is effective, it's mainly in slowing down tumors, rather than preventing them in the first place. If this is so, it means that selenium won't keep you from getting prostate cancer, but it might keep it from advancing.

To get at this definitively, the National Cancer Institutes have initiated a study called the Selenium and Vitamin E Cancer Prevent Trial (SELECT), which they bill as "the largest-ever prostate cancer prevention trial." They have 35,000 participants and began their work in earnest in the summer of 2004.

Vitamin E

Recently, the media have been pointing up a study that showed that large amounts of vitamin E supplements can be harmful. Smaller supplements can be useful in a wide variety of arenas, but proof about prostate cancer is not yet there. As always, check with your doctor before taking any supplements, especially if you're undergoing treatments.

Fish oils

For some years now, fish oil supplements (so-called EPA and DHA) have been touted as good for just about everything. Omega-3 fish oil is supposed to be helpful in a variety of health matters, ranging from depression to heart disease.

There is some evidence that omega-3 oils are also beneficial for prostate cancer. One study found that men who took 500 milligrams a day were 11 percent less likely to develop prostate cancer than men with an intake of less than 125 milligrams every day.

Again, this needs replication and verification, but since fish oil is available in fish, and since these supplements are not deemed to be harmful, if your doctor agrees, there is nothing wrong with taking fish oil supplements if someone is worried about contracting prostate cancer.

Foods that promote strength

I remember asking my doctor what I should eat when I was undergoing radiation. His answer was: a balanced diet. This is not quite what the NCI recommends. In fact, they say that how one eats just before and during treatment requires a different approach.

Balancing your foods and consuming low animal fats are not nearly as important, they say, as "higher calorie foods that emphasize protein." "Increasing your use of sauces and gravies, or changing cooking methods to include more butter or oil." And, with radiation, high-fiber foods—normally recommended for a healthy diet—might cause diarrhea when undergoing radiation to the prostate.

The idea is to increase your strength during treatment, which otherwise may lessen due to the radiation or other therapies. The goal—say the NCI—is to keep you eating, to keep tissue from breaking down, to "maintain defenses against infection."

Many people don't feel as hungry when they're under treatment. Nutrients have to keep pouring into your body. Eating enough is more important than worrying about balance, if you have little or no appetite. "Eat what you like," seems to be the dictum, and that way most men are likely to get enough protein and calories, which give strength.

What foods will lessen side effects?

It's not so much that specific foods or pills can lessen side effects, as that having a strong body can make you less susceptible to deleterious effects of radiation or surgery.

But in addition to eating well, the NCI suggests something very interesting. "Think positively," they say. Since you don't know whether you'll have any side effects, assume you won't. Being positive, talking about your worries, staying well-informed, reducing your anxiety level—all of these will, according to the NIC, help you stay more in control and reduce your side effects, not to mention increasing your appetite!

IN A SENTENCE:

> *No miracle food can cure cancer, but the right foods will help keep your body strong as you treat the cancer.*

living

What Prostate Cancer Isn't

ON DAY ONE, some of the symptoms of what *might be* prostate cancer were listed. As you'll recall, they were:

- ○ A flow of urine that stops and then goes, then stops again.
- ○ Having to get up in the night to urinate very often.
- ○ Painful urination.
- ○ Pain when you have an orgasm.
- ○ Urine that contains blood.
- ○ Persistent pain in and around the pelvic area, front or back.

But you'll also remember that most prostate cancer is discovered without these symptoms being present, and that these symptoms—if you look at them carefully—could be the result of numerous other—more serious, or more benign—physical changes in your body.

For instance, you can have pain urinating when you have a bladder infection—something easily treated with antibiotics. You can have frequent urination from infection, from BPH, from anxiety, or from a bladder that's lost its elasticity.

Blood in your urine can come from dangerous ailments such as bladder cancer and more benign ones such as high blood pressure. Kidney cancer, polycystic kidney disease, or simple urinary tract infection can also cause blood to seep into your urine.

And, you can have pain in the pelvic area from a kidney stone—one of the more painful events in anyone's life, but not life-threatening.

Medical students' syndrome

What happens when you learn a lot about any disease—as every medical student knows—is that you think you *have* that disease. So the twinge in your gut that could be anything from a hernia to too many *ab* exercises to indigestion becomes, in your mind, stomach or prostate cancer . . . or worse!

Stop!

You are not a diagnostician. You are not dying. Just as we have talked about the fact that prostate cancer is probably not going to kill you, you have to learn that symptoms—not even symptoms: what you *think* are symptoms—are not evidence of further disease.

If you have worries, by all means, look up the twinges or pain or discomfort or urinary blood in your Merck Manual (a medical students' guide that is now out in a lay version.) Sure, that could have the adverse effect of showing you all the terrible things the symptoms *could* be, but, more likely, will show you that your worries are inconsistent with anything serious. The manual may even guide you toward recognizing that some other condition than prostate cancer needs attending to.

If the symptoms persist, worsen, or still frighten you, call your physician, and let him interpret them.

Why is this happening . . . you're not a hypochrondriac!

You are not going crazy; your fears are not totally unfounded. What has happened is, your mind and your body have now become alert to the *reality* that you are not invulnerable, and to the *possibility* that terrible things can happen to you. That means you now find yourself hypersensitive to a lot of things that were entirely normal to your body previously, and that aren't signs of any kind of underlying ailment whatsoever. It's like buying a Volvo, and suddenly noticing that kind of car everywhere on the street. My God, you never saw so many Volvos before! Now, you're seeing signs of prostate cancer—or worse—throughout your body.

I'll give you two examples from my own experience.

Forgetting there are ordinary causes for ordinary ailments

Shortly after I had been diagnosed with lymphoma fifteen years ago—for which I received radiation treatment for twenty days and went into a remission that has lasted and lasted and lasted—I noticed a large lump in my arm, between my elbow and hand. I panicked. I was convinced that the cancer was back . . . and so soon after treatment, too. I phoned my oncologist and got an appointment for the next day. I didn't sleep that night. All the terrors of what I knew about the disease came flooding back. At my appointment, I waited three hours to see my doctor (he had squeezed me in to a busy day's schedule.) When he came in, he took one look and said, "Oh, didn't I tell you, there are no lymph nodes between the elbow and the hand." The bump turned out to be a hematoma from some heavy hammering I'd done the day before it appeared. So much for being hypersensitive . . . I'd been so focused on cancer that I'd tuned out any other reasonable cause for the lump. Now I have to face my oncologist's opening line whenever I return for a follow-up visit: "Any lumps or bumps?"

Remember: cancer treatment does not cure or prevent everything

From time to time, as we get older, small moles or other marks appear on our face or body. It's one of those things that keeps the cosmetic industry purring. Ever since I was diagnosed with cancer, years ago, my wife looks at these marks in a different way than she did previously. "Is that one growing?" "What's *that*?" "Are you sure you asked Dr. X about this one?" I am not anxious about these. But my wife is.

And perhaps she should be: Of course, the possibility that a mole might become skin cancer is totally unrelated to whether I ever had any other kind of cancer. It's a whole other kind of cancer, one that everyone should know the signs of even if they have never even had prostate cancer.

Being treated for prostate cancer doesn't mean you will never become ill from another disease. You may still come down with that bug going around your office; and obviously any other health problem you may already have or that may develop with age, such as diabetes, still needs to be attended to regardless of your treatment for prostate cancer.

Do you have to be careful not to "excite" the cancer?

The flip side of this is that it is unlikely you are going to do anything to yourself that could make the cancer "worse." Overeating at a holiday function, having a few drinks too many, getting the flu, whatever . . . they might make you feel bad in other ways, for sure, but will not cause the prostate cancer cells to grow any differently than they would otherwise. So while I'm not promoting overindulgence, neither should you be terrified of an occasional lapse. A night of wild sex, if you feel up to it, may exhaust you but won't hurt you. And, yes, you are still going to catch colds, pull muscles, and so on.

The treatment that may be eliminating your cancer does not make you invincible from everyday ailments. Just recognize other symptoms for what they are—they aren't cancer.

Is your immune system weakened by treatment?

One other thing. Unlike chemotherapy, or other kinds of strong medication, radiation does not necessarily render your immune system less able to function. Surgery *may* lay you up temporarily and require slow acceleration back to normal, and radiation *may* make you tired for a while; your immune system is up and running all the while. Unless your prostate cancer has progressed considerably, you are unlikely to have any serious side effects from these treatments (the few there are, are discussed in Week Four.)

A balanced outlook

If you feel lousy or tired or see lumps and bumps, take a few moments to explore the situation . . . then go on with your usual daily life. While you should stay alert to the possibility of other disorders as well as to a change in your own cancer—at the same time, avoid being *hyper*vigilant, because that can ruin your enjoyment of what is likely to be a long healthy life.

No, you aren't going to ever forget that you have prostate cancer. But you *can* learn to ignore the psychological and physical aftereffects of treatment, and pull back from becoming so knowledgeable about the illness itself that you see it at every turn.

IN A SENTENCE:

> *Don't be suspicious of every change in your body: not every symptom signifies cancer.*

learning

Preparing for the Worst while Hoping for the Best

What does the "worst" mean?

It's time to talk about worst-case scenarios. Not because I want to, but because you will probably want to—or your partner or wife may want to.

Oncologists don't like to talk about bad outcomes; indeed, most physicians don't like to.

Because (in their mind), it means they've "failed." It means that they can't do what they were trained to do: save lives, make people healthy.

What kind of bad outcomes am I talking about?

○ The cancer doesn't respond to the treatment.
○ You have a serious problem from the surgery or the anesthesia.
○ You have serious side effects.
○ Your prostate cancer metastasizes and is no longer treatable—this is unlikely for 85 to 90 percent of men with prostate cancer, but for the other 10 to 15 percent, it is possible.

I don't like to think about things like that. No one likes to think about things like that. But now is the time to do so. Because later, if something goes wrong, you may not be able to make or voice the kinds of decisions you would want to make.

If, for instance, you went into a coma during your surgery, or reacted very badly to the therapy in your clinical trial and couldn't communicate with anyone, your wife or partner may not know what to do next.

These include such decisions as:

○ How aggressively you would want the hospital to act to treat your pain.

○ Whether you would want to be put on a breathing machine if you couldn't breathe on your own.

These are the kinds of decisions we think of as associated with a terminal illness, not a chronic one, which is basically what prostate cancer is. But things can get out of control. Bad things happen to good people. So what you need to do, if you have not already done so, is take some steps to ensure that those closest to you, your medical team, and your lawyer know where you stand on the above decisions, and also on how you may wish your financial and other responsibilities handled if you are suddenly out of commission.

Living wills

You have undoubtedly heard about the legal entity called a living will. That's a document that allows you to state in fairly general terms what you do and do not want done about your health care or other matters should you become unable to communicate.

There are sample boilerplate living wills in books about health care and on the Internet. Or, using them as a model, you can write your own from scratch. Put into writing, in advance of your needs, what your feelings are about standard medical procedures, should you become unable to think or communicate clearly.

The health-care proxy

The health-care power of attorney (sometimes called "proxy") is another document that appoints someone (your "agent") to make specifically health-related choices for you, should you be unable to do so. This is a more powerful—and more flexible—document because you have chosen someone to actually be there to listen to and help the medical team decide what is best for you.

While hospitals and physicians are now required to ask you if you have such documents, millions of Americans haven't made out a living will, nor have they chosen a health-care agent.

This is not a good thing. In fact, having written a book about these matters, I believe anyone over fifty who doesn't have a living will and a proxy is making a big mistake.[1]

Having someone you trust, who can make decisions when you're in a coma—or even briefly daffy from too much pain medication—is a wonderful relief to people who have been through that. You don't have to be dying to use an agent. There may be any manner of times when you're temporarily out of it, and when the agent can and should step in.

An agent's job is to look to your wishes, whatever they may be. When the time comes, your agent will consult with physicians, clergy, social workers, and family members about your care, but in the end, the decision should be the agent's, acting as he or she believes you would want.

How do you choose such an agent?

First of all, this has to be a person whom you absolutely trust to carry out what you wish, someone who would put aside his or her preferences and values to honor yours.

Second, it has to be a person who will be available physically when you need him to be. In other words, someone who lives nearby. In fact, if you divide your life between two regions—say, Florida in the winter and farther north the rest of the year—it may be useful to appoint two agents, each respective to each region. Besides which, some U.S. states may not accept a power of attorney form not written and notarized within that state, so even if you have created such a form, it wouldn't hurt to write up a new one if you have since moved out of the state where it was written.

Third, this person has to be educated about your health care, your particular needs, and your particular wishes. How aggressive do you want the doctors to be if you are too woozy from medication to give an informed consent? What if you temporarily need help breathing, or a feeding tube. What if you're unconscious when such decisions need to be made? Your well-informed agent can make those decisions for you. And you can rescind them if you wish when you are able to think clearly and communicate.

So, you'll want to choose a person who is able to work with physicians, but not give in to their wishes. Someone who can really understand your needs, but has the gumption to hold on to his or her opinion when talking with you—so you can have a foil to discuss these things with.

Your wishes are going to change, so you'll want to have someone you can reach, can check in with, from time to time to convey your new ideas about what you do or don't want in terms of care when you can't make that decision yourself, or can't communicate it.

A lot of people choose their spouse or partner. That works sometimes, but other times it doesn't. My wife has chosen my youngest daughter to be her proxy. She's a lawyer; she'll be around when my wife gets a lot older (I may not be); and she's loving but tough!

I would next sit down with that person—before you decide for sure who you want—and talk with them about your ideas about care. Be as specific as you can in this discussion:

- ○ Where do you want to die—at home or in a hospital?
- ○ What kind of emergency equipment or interventions do you want? A lot of men want "everything" done for them to keep them alive, but until you've actually sat down and talked about each one of those eventualities, you really won't know how you feel.
- ○ Do you know enough about hospice and home care? If not, you and your agent should investigate possible facilities and services, and discuss them.
- ○ How do you feel about pain medication? How much do you want?
- ○ Do you have long-term care insurance? If not, why not? Investigate and make a decision. For most of us, Medicare won't pay for our needs if we're incapacitated but living at home; and many people have enough assets that Medicaid won't kick in. The only other option to pay for long-term care at home or in a nursing home is insurance. Yes, you don't want to think about such things, but now is the time to do that.
- ○ Finally, discuss your spiritual and emotional wishes with your agent. Some men and women don't want a rabbi or priest near them when they're ill. Others do, but don't think to specify this in advance.

After one or more such discussions, you'll get a feeling whether this person understands your wishes and will indeed carry them out.

If not, choose someone else. And don't be afraid, as the years go by, to change to someone else if need be.

Most people find that when they get into talking about these matters, little details get in the way. And it is often in the details that the distinction between comfort and discomfort lies.

And While You're At It . . .

COMPOSING A living will and choosing a health-care representative may cause you to think about some other issues you haven't addressed, such as who might run your business in your absence or whether your wife or someone else, such as your lawyer or accountant, knows enough about the family finances to take over dealing with such matters if you are incapacitated. If you have always handled such things yourself, you'd be surprised to know how many things like where you keep your extra checkbooks, or what projects need follow-up in your business, may be confusing to anyone else suddenly needing to take over such matters. How much or how little you care to spell out is up to you, but let's put it this way: you don't want to come home from the hospital, or whatever, and find your affairs in a mess because you never instructed anyone else about what to do. This is not the time to be secretive or egocentric. Write down what may need to be done and where important things are kept. Be sure that the person or people who will need to refer to the document have a copy or will know where to obtain it in an emergency.

IN A SENTENCE:

Even if you think you may not need them, creating a living will and appointing a health-care rep will give you and your loved ones peace of mind.

living

Six-Month Checkup

What to expect and learn from your checkups

When you get your first checkup depends on the kind of treatment you've had.

But that doesn't change the words your doctor will use. The terms "three-month checkup" and "six-month checkup" are meant to imply a periodic checking up on your condition, and whether they actually come at precisely three or six months after treatment is not important. What is important is that your oncologist will first want to see you every three months for a while, then every six months and, finally, once a year.

So, I will treat the six-month checkup as emblematic of all your checkups.

Any visit to your oncologist is an opportunity to do a variety of things, some of which will be initiated by him, and some initiated by you. During the waiting period between checkups, you may think—or wish—that you had heard from him. I know that I did, and I thought, "Gee, I'm a prized patient of this doctor. Why doesn't he call?" He's too busy, that's why. Use the hiatus to compose a list of questions to ask him, or other matters you feel the need to discuss with him, issues that are not so urgent that you need to make a special call before the checkup date and yet important enough that you want to remember to bring them up when the time comes.

What will your doctor check?

Your oncologist will schedule some tests, perhaps at a lab, just as you did for your initial diagnosis. You'll have a blood test, including a PSA. That may be it. If your PSA has decreased by more than 1 or 2 points, that's good. If it was very high to begin with, and it's gone down 4 or 5 points, that's even better.

If you are a Stage III patient, more tests will be done. You may have a follow-up CAT scan or MRI or X-ray to determine shrinkage of your tumors.

If you are a Stage IV patient, you can be sure that you'll have advanced tests to see where things stand.

When you arrive in the examining room, the doctor's nurse or assistant will ask a series of questions, such as:

○ Are you eating your regular diet?
○ Have you had any bleeding through your anus or when you urinate?
○ Any pain when you urinate?
○ Do you have an "urgent" need to urinate from time to time?
○ How is your sexual activity? Do you have any pain when you ejaculate?
○ How is your bladder and bowel control?
○ Do you sleep well? Are you fatigued?
○ Any eating problems?
○ Any sore throats, infections?
○ Any skin problems?

You'll have your blood pressure taken, and your temperature.

Then, you'll see the doctor. He'll have the answers to your questions, and will ask you about any irregularities in them. He'll do a DRE. If your prostate has shrunk, he'll consider that a good sign.

If you've had surgery, the doctor will check your scars and make sure everything is healing.

And if you're a Stage II or Stage III patient, the doctor will discuss with you where things stand according to your latest test results. This may be good news, bad news, or no news at all.

If you're a late-stage patient, your physician may also suggest a colonoscopy. The idea here is to examine the entire length of your colon, otherwise known as the intestine, which terminates at the upper end at your stomach, with the lower end at your rectum. If you have had cancer cells migrate from the prostate, some of them may have made it into the colon. Within a short time (maybe two hours), a specialist can determine the facts.

What you need to do

You need to take this time to ask about anything that bothers you at present or concerns you about the future.

The doctors are so used to seeing dozens of patients, and so used to having the treatments "work," that they see these sessions as routine. Unless something shows up in the blood tests or CAT scans, they want to get in and out as quickly as possible, to move on to the patient who hasn't been seen yet.

But this is your only time, until your next checkup, to be face-to-face with your doctor and get some direct answers to what you may have noted on that list I spoke about. Some answers may be predictable but ask anyway.

For instance:

- Is this pain in my rectum ever going to go away? [Most likely he'll say, if it doesn't, call me, and we'll see what's going on.]
- I haven't had any sign of incontinence yet; does that mean I won't have any? [Probably.]
- I find I suddenly need to go to the bathroom, then can't urinate. Does that mean anything serious? [No. It's quite expected after most treatments.]
- I tried Viagra. It doesn't work. [Make sure you take it on an empty stomach. Before dinner, say. And then forget about it. Let nature take its course. Or, keep trying for a while. If that doesn't work, we'll talk about alternatives.]

Dealing with bad news

It would be lovely to assume that your checkups will always be good ones. It would be wonderful if you got to your oncologist and he looked at your PSA level and did a DRE and said, "Everything's going fine."

It doesn't always happen.

You may report a little blood in your urine or stool. You may feel tired, more tired than you were three months ago. Your PSA may even have gone up a little. Your doctor may suggest that you come back in three months, rather than after the six-month interval he'd led you to believe was "normal."

A lot of this will really depend on three things:

○ What kind of treatment you had. If you had surgery, you can expect a longer recovery time and, perhaps, some unpleasant aftereffects which last or surface at this time. If you've had seed implants or radiation, probably not, but always possible.

○ What your mind-set is. Some people, including myself, approach these checkups with trepidation. Anxiety and depression can show themselves as lethargy, pain in the stomach, headaches—you name it. This can indicate anxiety and depression, *not* progress of the disease. So, while your cancer is actually under control, your doctor may wish to see you again sooner or send you to a specialist to treat these associated issues.

○ The disease process itself. Yes, it's possible that your disease may have returned. It's more likely at six months that you are simply experiencing benign side effects that may have kicked in at some delay following your treatment. In fact, for most Stage I to II prostate cancer, it's *highly unlikely* that your tumor would recur in such a short time. Highly unlikely.

So, if your oncologist remarks upon your PSA or feels "something" in your prostate, do not panic. It's most likely to be an anomaly that he—being the good physician he is—will want to keep tabs on it. That's all.

Go on about your life, knowing that recovery, like everything else in the world of health and medicine, is not a straight-line phenomenon, but knowing, too, that you are most likely on the road to a smooth, uneventful rise from a relatively minor process. Unless you have been diagnosed in Stage III or Stage IV, you are, most likely, now healthy at the six-month point. Does that mean you *never* need to go back? Absolutely not. Read on.

Keep going to your checkups

There may be a tendency on your part to think that checkups are a waste of time. Especially if you've had seed implantation or external radiation, and all your side effects have disappeared—or almost; you may think it's something you no longer need to do. Why?

○ Because you are sure you're cured
○ Because you don't like being reminded that you have cancer
○ Because you worry for three or four weeks before each checkup

My first checkup

Here's how I felt when I went for my first checkup.

I went to the hospital to meet with B. After my usual forty-five-minute wait in a cold cubicle, he came in alone and asked, in his deadpan manner, whether I was feeling any side effects. "None, except the urination thing," I answered. He did a cursory check, pronounced me "Okay, as far as I can tell," and ordered me into the Blood Drawing room for some tests. They took four times the usual amount checking for all the little things that can show up after radiation. Then he told me I should come back in *three* months for more CAT scans.

I was shocked. I'd really put additional testing out of my mind. I didn't plan on needing anything more. The anxiety began again, creeping up into my chest. I didn't know if I could live like this—every six months having CAT scans, "just in case." There wasn't supposed to be any "just in case." Those thirty-five days of radiation were supposed to kill off the cells. Forever.

Dealing with checkup anxiety

There is no forever cure. Yes, even the most successful treatment means a future of perpetual worry. You're in this game for the rest of your life. Testing to see if there's another mysterious little cell somewhere.

You need the fact that, even years down the line, you may experience some emotional shudders as the checkup date approaches. You may become short-tempered and not know why. You may feel depressed and not know why. You may get a stomachache or diarrhea or even what resembles the flu, and not associate those ailments with anxiety over your next appointment. This is because the word "cancer" continues to reverberate in your mind, even if you're not aware of it.

It's been fifteen years since I got lymphoma, and four years since I had treatment for prostate cancer, and every appointment is still preceded by some unexpected physical or emotional upset.

This is not written to scare you. It is a way of pointing out that such inner turmoil is normal, and to some extent created by the same fight-or-flight adrenaline rush that you experienced at your initial diagnosis at the same facility or with the same oncologist. Most of these feelings are snarled in memories and "what ifs," not "what is."

As you anticipate your appointment, try to channel some of your attention and energy into surveying all the positive aspects of "what is." Along with queries and complaints you may have for your doctor, list for yourself, and then be sure to tell him, the kinds of progress you have made since he last saw you, such as your old appetite returning, or your having had the energy to take vacation with your family. He needs to know these things, too, even if he seems impatient to get on to the next patient. He needs to know whether you *feel* better, not just whether the tests say you are.

The likelihood is that those tests will turn up nothing negative; that once the checkup is over, you will have nothing to show for the visit except a pinprick where they took blood; irritation because your doctor didn't spend as much time as you would have liked with you; and a nagging feeling that this should be your last checkup because you're OK now.

Don't let anxiety or annoyance or bravado stand in the way of having regular checkups. Don't shirk your responsibility to yourself and your family.

Since there aren't yet any absolute guarantees of a cure, you need to continue to stay on top of your disease, even if to confirm that it has not returned or progressed. Your doctor is actually your ally in this, not an enemy.

So—take your appointments with good grace, and go to them. Think of them as an extra tool to measure and confirm your progress, not as a rendezvous with certain doom.

IN A SENTENCE:

> *Regular checkups are often a time to hear good news and to ask all the questions you need to ask.*

learning

Data on Treatment Results

ONE OF the first questions someone who is diagnosed with prostate cancer asks is, "What's the chance of my having a complete recovery?"

> When I finally got past my biopsy and the pathology report, I secured an appointment with the "top man" at a big hospital. He breezed into the tiny examination room and plopped himself down on a wheeled stool which allowed him to come up very close in my face. "So," he said, rather unctuously, "You want to be cured." A huge smile crossed his face.—SAMUEL H.

Samuel H. wasn't used to doctors who still behaved like Gods, and he didn't like it; not one bit. Actually, Samuel, like most of us, was willing to settle for something less than a cure. He just wanted to be treated so he wouldn't be in pain or die from this cancer.

Does that mean there is no cure?

The word "cure" is a strange one. Some oncologists won't use it at all. The doctor who sees to my lymphoma always talks about it as a "chronic disease," and talks in terms of "five years out." "Five years" is actually a very common term in the cancer field. Studies and prognosticators talk about "a person in such and such a condition will most likely get to the five-year mark with this and that treatment." This allows for a certain amount of latitude in **prognoses**. After that five-year mark, the physician may look to ten years out, and so on.

Let's talk about the data surrounding prostate cancer. I've been over some of this before, but it's worth looking at again, now that you've come partway down the road.

This is a common disease. Even if there are no symptoms, a microscope can detect cancerous cells in most men over fifty years old. If you add twenty-five years to that age—seventy-five—it's estimated that 75 percent of the male population actually has some cancer of the prostate. Yet only a small number of men are diagnosed with prostate cancer, and only a fraction of those elect to be treated for it. The current numbers are 230,000 cases a year (about 16 percent of American men), very few of whom will die from the disease—at this time, it works out to about 29,000 a year. That seems like a large number of people, but when compared with mortality rates of other cancers, it's actually quite good.

Here's how the stage of your cancer relates to your probable survival past five years:

○ If your cancer is totally within your prostate gland, it is highly likely that you will survive past five years.
○ If your cancer is outside, but near the gland, it's not considered "curable," though it is treatable, and while many men with this "locally advanced cancer" will die of the disease, it's also possible that you will live more than five years.
○ The news is not good for prostate cancer patients whose malignant cells have metastasized to distant organs and the bones. It cannot be cured, though it can be slowed down. Survival is one to three years. Remember, at present this group is only 11 percent of those who have been diagnosed with prostate cancer. And the NCI says that "Even in this group of patients, [patients] have lived for many years."

One Study

IN ONE study, doctors tracked for over eight years nearly two hundred men with high-risk prostate cancer, to see if adding external-beam radiation and hormone therapy to brachytherapy did indeed increase disease-free survival rates.

Of the participating patients, 107 men were treated with external-beam radiation therapy combined with seed implants. Another 69 patients received hormone therapy in addition to the seed implants and external-beam radiation. After eight years, nearly 94 percent of the men who had hormone therapy in addition to the two types of radiation had no evidence of their prostate cancer, compared with 84 percent of the men who only had seed implants and external beam radiation therapy.

"This is an exciting study because it shows that adding hormone treatment and external beam radiation therapy to seed implants does indeed help men with high-risk prostate cancer to live longer without the cancer returning," said Gregory S. Merrick, MD, lead author of the study.

Mortality

Looking at the inverse of survival—mortality, researching very specific rates of death from prostate cancer in any one locality is not easy. I did find this data from Olmsted County, Minnesota. The report from which this data comes sheds some light also on the question of what is known or not known about the variable death rate and its relationship to the PSA screening.

Prostate cancer mortality rates increased from 25.8 per 100,000 men in the population during the period 1980 to 1984 to a peak of 34 per 100,000 during 1989 to 1992; they subsequently decreased to 19.4 per 100,000 during 1993 to 1997. Similar observations have been made elsewhere in the world, leading some to hypothesize that the mortality decline is related to PSA testing. In Canada (Quebec province), however, examinations of the association between the size of the decrease in mortality rates (from 1995 to 1999), suggests that, at least over this time frame, the decline in mortality is not related to widespread PSA testing. Cause-of-death misclassification has also been studied as a possible explanation for changes in prostate cancer mortality.

Recurrence

The NCI has this to offer about the likelihood of cancer returning:

One study followed two thousand men who had had radical prostatectomies. Three hundred and fifteen men were examined because their PSA levels rose some time after the operations. Of these, only one hundred men showed evidence of recurrence of cancer. It took an average eight years for metastatic cancer to emerge as the PSA went up again; and after that, the average time before death was another five years. Looked at from another point of view—that seems to mean that up to thirteen years of life past their operations existed for those men whose cancer eventually returned and metastasized.

For those who had radiation, seed implantation, and other of the newer treatments, no current data on survival is stable enough to deliver.

How to interpret all this

The chance of your prostate cancer becoming serious (i.e., spreading and causing major health problems) depends on the stage of your cancer, your age, your general health, the Gleason score, and how long you've had it.

Early in this book, I talked about the differentiation of cancer cells. If the cells are "well-differentiated," in their own locatable clumps, they are less likely to be serious cancer than if they are chaotic, or scattered in many places. That's one of the things that determines whether you have a low or a high Gleason. If you have a relatively low Gleason (1 to 4) and your cancer is within the prostate gland itself, scientists say that, with or without treatment, your five-year outcome is pretty damn good. So is your ten-year outcome. I mean by that: if you are Stage I and have a low Gleason, you aren't likely to have died from prostate cancer when ten years have gone by.

Let's repeat that, with a slightly different emphasis: If you are in a low-ranking stage and have treatment of any kind—and that means watchful waiting, not necessarily surgery or radiation—you will be 80 to 90 percent certain of dying of something other than prostate cancer.

Here is some additional encouraging information summing up what is known at present:

○ Based on cases diagnosed in 1990 and followed through 1995, 93 percent of all men diagnosed with prostate cancer survive five years or longer.
○ Relative survival rates have increased since 1973 for both black and white men, but the difference between blacks and whites has increased over time (survival has not improved as rapidly in black men).
○ The survival rate has increased over time for all grades of cancer.

And two downers:

○ The survival rate for younger men (under fifty) is lower than for older men.
○ Survival for cancer that has spread has not improved; five-year survival for that kind of cancer is only 34 percent.

Let's look at this analysis again in a different format. Some people find it easier to understand such information when it is presented as a table.

If your prostate cancer is ...	Your chance of surviving 5 years is ...
Stage I or Stage II	96 percent
Stage III	74 percent
Stage IV	30 to 50 percent

And once more.

For those who find bar charts and graphs easy to read, the following are taken from the NCI's SEER program (Surveillance, Epidemiology, and End Results).

Prostate Cancer
SEER 5-Year and 10-Year Survival Rates, 1973–1990

Observed Survival Rates

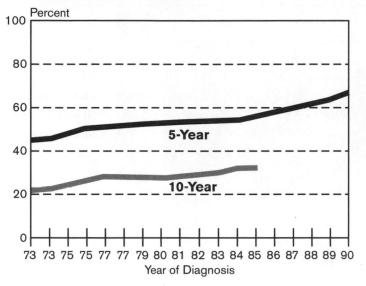

Relative Survival Rates

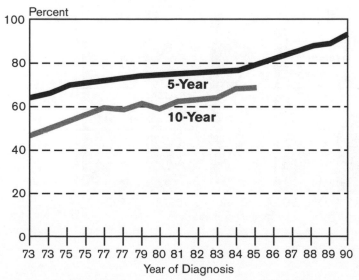

Prostate Cancer
SEER 5-Year Relative Survival Rates,
By Race

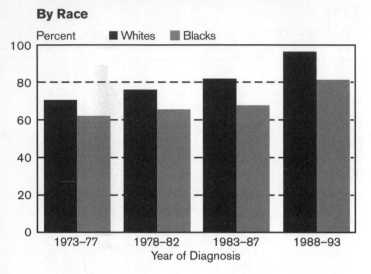

Percent ■ Whites ■ Blacks

Year of Diagnosis

By Age at Diagnosis

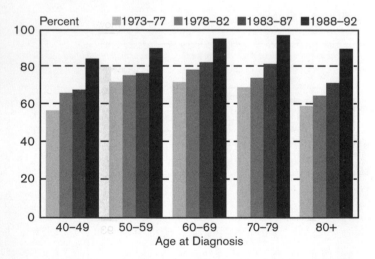

Percent ■1973–77 ■1978–82 ■1983–87 ■1988–92

Age at Diagnosis

Prostate Cancer
SEER 5-Year Relative Survival Rates,

By Stage

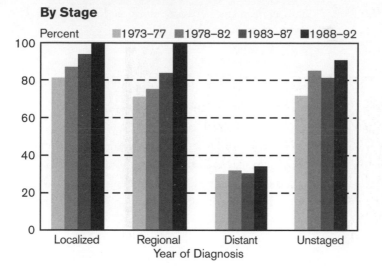

Percent ■1973–77 ■1978–82 ■1983–87 ■1988–92

Year of Diagnosis

(Localized, Regional, Distant, Unstaged)

By Grade

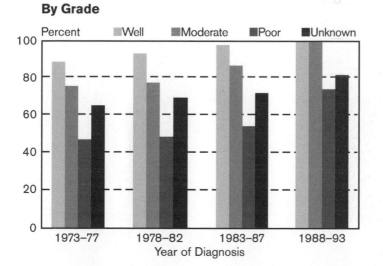

Percent ■Well ■Moderate ■Poor ■Unknown

Year of Diagnosis

(1973–77, 1978–82, 1983–87, 1988–93)

As with any data of this sort, what's true for a class of patients (for instance, all those diagnosed in 1989) may or may not be true for any individual. To put it in baldly, there aren't enough statistics right now to know if being treated for prostate cancer, and how you are treated, will make a difference in how long you survive.

What about stage IV cancer?

If your prostate cancer has spread to the nearby lymph nodes or to distant parts of the body, it is called metastatic prostate cancer. The outlook for men in Stage IV is not good. Hormonal therapy will generally improve your symptoms and delay the progress of disease for another two to three years. If just the lymph nodes are involved, a man may use hormonal therapy to delay the progress of prostate cancer even longer. However, the sad fact is that the vast majority of those with positive lymph nodes at the time of getting hormonal therapy will remain at risk of developing additional metastatic disease within ten years after the treatment. Bone metastases tend to be less responsive to hormonal therapy.

But, again, I hasten to add that not enough comparative studies have been done to discover whether aggressive cancer, once discovered, can be successfully stopped. Those studies are presently underway.

IN A SENTENCE:

Facts and figures are important, but can be very confusing.

HALF-YEAR MILESTONE

During the past six months, you have come a long way in your education about the physical and psychological effects of prostate cancer. Here are some things to keep in mind.

○ DECIDING ON TREATMENT FOR PROSTATE CANCER CAN BE DIFFICULT BECAUSE OF ALL THE OPINIONS AND THE AS-YET-UNDETERMINED PROOF THAT ONE OPTION WORKS BETTER THAN ANOTHER.

○ KEEPING UP YOUR HEALTH—THROUGH PHYSICAL EXERCISE AND PROPER EATING—CAN HELP FIGHT BOTH THE UNDERLYING CANCER AND YOUR TREATMENT REGIMEN.

○ YOU MAY NEED HELP IN FIGHTING TO GET YOUR TREATMENT PAID FOR, BUT IT CAN BE DONE.

○ IF YOUR CANCER REQUIRES SOMETHING SPECIAL, OR YOUR INSURER IS BALKING AT COVERING YOUR TREATMENT, LOOK INTO CLINICAL TRIALS.

○ IMPOTENCE CAN OCCUR WITH TREATMENT FOR PROSTATE CANCER. RESTORING YOUR SEXUAL LIFE WITH A PARTNER CAN BE

DONE—WITH EFFORT AND GOODWILL ON YOUR PART.

○ GETTING REGULAR CHECKUPS MAY BE HARD ON YOUR PSYCHE, BUT THEY'RE WORTH DOING.

○ DESPITE ALL THE UNKNOWNS ABOUT THIS DISEASE, MORE DATA WILL BECOME AVAILABLE ABOUT THE EFFICACY OF TREATMENT IN THE YEARS TO COME.

Resuming Sex

YOU HAVE refrained from sexual activity up until this time. The reasons for this may be:

○ You don't want to explore the possibility that you're partially impotent.

○ Someone in your medical team has cautioned you that sex might be painful.

○ You've discovered that it actually can be slightly painful when you have an orgasm and you don't want to go through that again.

○ Your wife or partner, in an effort to be careful of your physical and emotional well-being, doesn't make any overtures in this arena.

Whatever the reason, and there can be more, many men find it important to reassess their sexual activity at this time.

Age and sex

I have touched on this before, but I want to go into it again. It's important.

The myths about old age and sex start very young. Partly they come from an emphasis on youth and virility that we obtain in our early years and hold on to for our entire lives: that only young and beautiful bodies are made for sex. That just isn't true.

One Web site puts it this way:

> Although one's sex drive declines with age, the rate and the extent of this decline are often exaggerated. In fact, desire and capacity for intercourse are often retained into old age. Usually, fears of social disapproval, worries about not being attractive as before, or doubts about sexual performance may lead a couple to give up sexual activity prematurely.[1]

My parents? My grandparents?

As youngsters, even as we ourselves advance into middle age, it is often difficult to think of our parents having sex. Or even wanting to have sex. As for our grandparents—that's a stretch. We find such thoughts uncomfortable for some reason, even once we're at or past the age of our forebears.

It's only one of a number of "ageist" concepts that many people have. Those concepts contribute mightily to the perception that mature adults can't participate in sports, need to be forced into retirement at a set age, can't learn how to use a computer, and so forth. The myth we're concerned with now, of course, is that older people—male and female alike—don't retain sexual desire and pursue sexual activity.

Admittedly, for most of us, the desire is not always as exotic or exciting; the ability to perform in the same manner as in our youth is not always there; but there are many compensations and many pleasures awaiting people who continue sex into their oldest years.

What may change with age . . . or cancer

One of the unfortunate changes that may come with time is impotence. Even if he still has sexual desire, partial or total impotence will obviously play a role in preventing a man from engaging in intercourse. And this is even without the added problem of prostate cancer and its treatments.

Here's what one scholarly paper on the subject has to say:

Although the incidence of sexual dysfunction increases in old age, this is primarily related to the increased rate of health problems, rather than old age per se. Numerous endocrine, vascular, and neurological disorders may interfere in sexual function, as may many forms of medication and surgery. These health factors are more prevalent in older people and hence it is perhaps not surprising to find an increase in biologically caused sexual problems in the elderly.[2]

Women or partners may interpret the fact that a man is partially impotent as a sign of a lack of interest . . . in them, or in sex itself. That's too bad, because if the impotence is caused by some medical treatment, rather than his own reduced desire, there's nothing a man would rather do than have his old flair back again.

But, mark my word, the ability to enjoy lovemaking can continue well into old age, particularly if a couple make the effort to understand and respond to the various changes that age brings to the natural pattern of sexual response, such as a need for additional foreplay to become physically aroused. All too often, older people give up intercourse because they mistakenly interpret these changes as signs of impending impotence. It is important to recognize that one may also enjoy a lesser or incomplete degree of arousal, as both a physical outlet and an expression of emotional intimacy.

Sure, lovemaking may have to be a more leisurely affair as a couple gets older, but the benefits of maintaining the sexual aspect of the relationship into old age can be great. You can't assume that your wife or partner doesn't share your interest in it, or in fact may not have been experiencing some changes of her own that have given her a renewed desire for you:

In older women, the physiological effects of aging on sexual function are primarily caused by decreased amounts of circulating estrogen after menopause. The rate and amount of vaginal lubrication are decreased, and there is general atrophy of vaginal tissue. For many women, these changes associated with menopause are more than offset by the freedom to explore and enjoy sexual activity without the worry of becoming pregnant.

White (1982) reviewed the literature on sex and aging and concluded that sexual behavior and attitudes in old age reflect a continuation of lifelong patterns, hence those who are most sexually active in their younger years tend to continue this pattern in their later years. Negative attitudes toward sex learned at a young age may seriously impair the ability to enjoy sex in later life.[3]

Rethinking the connection when cancer enters the picture

As one man, Herman J., put it, "Marriages have to rethink the connection" when confronted with prostate cancer.

His wife, Charlotte, had a rather poignant remark about her husband's condition: "First, you're grateful for life; then you want more."

There are several means by which to recharge your sex life.

Sex therapy

You've seen those ads in the back of magazines. "Buy this book," "Buy this video," "Enjoy sex again." I really don't know what's in those books or videos. Soft pornography, I suspect. For those couples whose love bonds are still strong but whose sexual activity has diminished because of prostate cancer, a little soft porn isn't necessarily a bad thing. It can stimulate both partners to sexual activity they hadn't thought of or felt like in a while.

But to those for whom the idea of any kind of pornography is anathema, or who are too embarrassed to explore that world, there is a perfectly respectable line of approach. And that is sex therapy.

Sex therapists have been around a long time. They aren't just the far reaches of the sexual revolution of the 1960s and '70s, or an outreach effort of the Kinsey Report. They are a bona fide branch of psychology, which explores why couples don't enjoy each other sexually as much as they either used to or wish they could, and what to do about it.

The most typical technique in sex therapy—after a discussion with the therapist about wishes, problems, and any prior experience with therapy—is what might be called "sensual touching." This involves nothing more than "homework" for a couple, in which they are instructed not to try for sexual activity but to refrain from it, in favor of simply touching each other's body—arms, face—to reacquaint themselves with the other person and their own pleasure in a *sensual*, but not necessarily *sexual* way. Massage over a long period of time can also be helpful.

One of the things this process does is, it takes the pressure off having sex as a goal in and of itself. By telling a couple not to have sex, but simply to explore each other's body, neither partner feels guilty or embarrassed about not feeling "up to it," and may in fact discover new ways of engaging with each other that they will enjoy continuing even if and when sex is resumed.

There are some rather questionable ads in periodicals or sites on the Net. My own feeling is that this is not something you want to do over the phone or via Internet. You want to meet a qualified sex therapist face-to-face, get a feeling for his or her ethics and personality. You want to enter into this without a feeling of shame. A very good introduction to sex therapy and sex therapists can be found on the Internet at http://coolnurse.healthology.com/webcast_transcript.asp.

Many books on this subject could enable you and your partner to explore kinds of touching and even sexual positions that you may not have considered before, without bringing a third person into the bed with you, so to speak. There is good reason to persist—for both of you. Recent laboratory experiments have shown that the chemical oxytocin is released when humans touch each other. This is the same chemical that is released when illegal drugs are used—though not in the same amount. It has been nicknamed the "cuddle chemical," because it can be released with just the stroking of the skin, and thus plays a role in maintaining love between married couples. It "deepens tenderness between familiar partners," is the way one researcher put it.[4]

The point is, if you have not already realized this already, now is the time to appreciate that lovemaking does not always have to culminate in intercourse. That can be an incredibly liberating mind-set for both parties in a relationship, well into very old age.

Your medical team

Unfortunately, it's not easy to talk with others about sex and, sad to say, most health-care professionals aren't trained to talk about it. If you want to, however, your doctor and other staff you have become familiar with during treatment are not a bad place to start.

So, start by talking to your oncologist, a member of his team (including the nurses), or your personal physician.

If that doesn't get you anywhere, ask for a referral to someone who specializes in sexual problems. Ask around your hospital or cancer care institution. There is going to be someone associated with your treatment, who has expertise in this arena. There may even be a support group for sexual problems at nearby hospitals, though you will most likely have had to be treated there to take advantage of that program.

Another place to consider getting help are stand-alone "sex clinics," or clinics associated with medical schools. These, too, can be very helpful, and your doctor(s) may be able to place you. Again, though, it's important to find a reputable and experienced group of personnel. Take your time finding the right one for you and your partner.

You might also want to look up branches of the American Association of Sex Educators, Counselors, and Therapists (AASECT) at www.aasect.org, which can at least tell you who in your town belongs to this organization, and therefore who is licensed and practiced.

Finally, try any of the social workers or psychologists in your neighborhood. Even though they may not practice sex therapy or be members of a clinic, they may have colleagues who are.

And don't forget your feelings

In other chapters we have dealt at some length on obtaining psychotherapy or counseling if you are anxious or depressed. Impotence and the mental pain it causes to both partners in a relationship are prime causes of depression after treatment for prostate cancer. Don't forget to go back to anyone who has given you psychological help in this health battle—see what they can do for you now. Even if they are unable to solve a physical problem you are experiencing, they can assist you in how you deal with it emotionally.

What not to do

The American Cancer Society suggests that it would be unwise to try the following kinds of "solutions" to your sexual problems: "Potency pills, such as poppers or Spanish fly, oysters, hypnotism by someone not trained as a mental health professional, a sexual surrogate."

IN A SENTENCE:

> *If lovemaking was important to you before you got prostate cancer, it can remain important now.*

learning

Pain Control

Pain with stage I or II prostate cancer

The likelihood of having pain with these low stage cancers is very slight. When you have treatment, there will be the usual discomfort arising from the form of treatment you choose. With surgery, there will be incisions and stitches; and the recovery time from them, while short, will include some pain. However, normal **analgesics** can probably handle that pain.

If not, let me repeat what I said in Week Four about minor pain relief. You can try:

○ Professional massage
○ Home massage
○ TENS machine
○ Heating pad
○ Cold packs
○ Acupuncture
○ Biofeedback

For postsurgery pain in your groin or in the anus or rectum, a remarkably effective and soothing remedy can be the old-fashioned warm bath. Sitting in a tub of hot water (not too hot!) can relax muscles and ease moderate pain.

With radiation, there is no pain from the treatment. After a session, you may experience several kinds of discomfort, the worst of which will most likely be a stinging sensation in the underside of your penis after an orgasm. You will have to decide whether it is worth having sex if it results in such discomfort, but most men I talked to said that it was worth it.

A word of caution, however. Your partner may be disturbed by your pain to the extent that she (or he) may hold back during sex or feel reluctant to engage in it, for fear of hurting you. One man told me that his wife was so upset that he had any pain that she didn't want to have sex at all. It took some doing on his part to persuade her it was worth it to him.

This postradiation pain may lessen as the months and years go by. Many say it does.

Pain with metastatic cancer

When prostate cancer spreads, either into the bones or into other organs, eventually it will cause some pain and other symptoms. You may become tired, you may lose weight. Cancer in the bones can be very debilitating.

The normal course of action for metastatic cancer is, as we have said, hormone therapy. This often reduces the size of the tumors, and that alone will help to relieve any pain you might be feeling. Radiation can also be useful in reducing the size of tumors, if the cancer is in identifiable and small enough areas. You don't want to have radiation over large areas of your body, but radiation into your bones—where pain is especially great—cannot only relieve the pain but slow down the growth of the cancer.

Unfortunately, hormone therapy stops working after a while. Your body—and your cancer—doesn't react positively anymore. The tumors will grow and additional radiation will not make them shrink. The pain can return.

And, unfortunately, only so much radiation can be given to any one patient before harm occurs, in the form of damaged tissue, bone, and organs.

The NCI makes clear that there are other options, however, including steroids. And there are always opioids—morphinelike painkillers.

Palliative care

For too many decades, physicians have been undermedicating pain. The fear that patients might become addicted to narcotic-type drugs—

morphine being the primary one—kept them from giving the increasingly sophisticated drugs to patients in sufficient amounts to truly reduce or eliminate their pain. And they tended to wait to administer painkillers until a patient was truly in agony.

A more enlightened approach has gradually taken over. Pain has been added to the critical list of questions that are asked of patients when they enter a hospital, have treatment or surgery, or when they have a serious ailment. A scale of 1 to 10 is used, and little faces (ranging from smiles to serious frowns) accompany those numbers. If you've been in a hospital recently, you'll recognize the pattern: they take your temperature, take your blood pressure, weigh you, and ask whether you have any pain. The next step, if you indicate you are experiencing pain, is deciding what to do about it . . . including if you indicate a lower number on the scale.

Over the years, doctors and nurses in hospices discovered one crucial fact: unless a person was already addicted, it was highly unlikely that the use of opiate-type drugs to relieve physical pain would make him an addict. This resulted in a revolution in treating pain, the beginning of a whole new movement, called palliative care, and relief for tens of thousands of patients.

When I was in the hospital for a resection of my colon—an operation that was done with tiny incisions—I experienced a lot of pain. For several days. While I lay in bed, I was hooked up to a pump that gave me a jolt of morphinelike substance every twenty minutes. If I needed more, I could push a button and receive one or two additional doses.

This kept ahead of the pain, treating it before it could become intense. Keeping ahead of pain is one key means of using less medication and having less pain. It has taken many years for the medical community to discover this fact, and it will take a decade or more before all practitioners accept this, but it is standard practice now in most modern hospitals to follow this model of pain control.

You may recall a vivid example of this when the Ukrainian opposition candidate Yushenko was poisoned by dioxin. His Viennese doctors put a pump under his skin so that he could have a morphine derivative go directly to his spinal cord, killing the devastating pain in his back. If the painkiller had gone into his veins, it would have affected his ability to think and talk, perhaps even walk, as it would go directly into his brain. But this way, it went where it was needed, and he could function. And get elected.

But what if you are not in the hospital?

Unhospitalized patients may also use morphine substitutes, which are available by prescription. These include such painkillers as Codeine, Fentanyl, Hydromorphone, Levorphanol, Methadone, Meperidine, Oxycontin, Oxymorphone, Percocet, and Vicodin, all related chemically to Oxycodone, or morphine. Don't stint. If your physician tells you it's safe to take three or four Percocet a day, do so. Palliative care specialists assert that all but a tiny (maybe 5 percent) of cancer patients with even the worst pain can be helped to get that pain under control. Living in pain puts extra stress upon your entire system; don't insist on braving it out without help.[5]

What about side effects?

Yushenko and his doctors knew about possible side effects from heavy doses of morphine, and worked around them. My own experience was a little different. After a couple of days in the hospital, after my operation, I began to realize that I was overmedicated from the pump. I wasn't addicted, I was just woozy and fuzzy. I couldn't see very well; I could not talk very well. I was, well, high! I asked them to discontinue the pump and to give me pills that I could take when I felt pain might be coming on. This way I got a lesser dose, but I still contained the pain.

Some people experience nausea or dizziness with opioids. If you have trouble with injections or the pump, or with taking pills, you can also get these drugs through skin patches.

What the national institute for cancer has to say about pain medications

The NIC has a very good Web site section on pain. Go to the main site, then look for a sidebar that says, "General Cancer Library." You'll find there a section called "Coping with Cancer." Look for "Pain" and you'll find pages on the subject, some of which applies to prostate cancer, but all of which applies to life!

Below, I've summarized some of this section for your use:

○ Don't feel you have to rely only on over-the-counter medicines like aspirin, though they're not a bad place to start when pain threatens.

○ Do consult with your health-care providers about your pain. They may have knowledge about new drugs that work, or old ones that don't. Besides, you'll need their prescriptions for those that are not over the counter.

○ Severe pain can be blocked by surgery or by injecting medicine directly into the nerves.

○ For those very few people for whom opioids and other techniques don't work, some may turn to conventional therapies or professional hypnosis to relieve pain. Another thing to think about is that pain makes people very unhappy. Depression and irritation, anger and despair are all part of the pain package. A therapist can help calm you down, even as the pain persists.

○ Do not be embarrassed or afraid to describe your pain in detail to your health-care professionals. You are not a sissy because you have pain. Pain is real. Pain is a terrible thing to undergo. It is your right to seek pain relief.

○ Once you start taking pain medication, make sure you get the right and most complete information about what has been prescribed for you.

The NCI says to ask:

○ How much medicine should I take? How often?

○ If my pain is not relieved, can I take more? If the dose should be increased, by how much?

○ Should I call you before increasing the dose?

○ What if I forget to take it or take it too late?

○ Should I take my medicine with food?

○ How much liquid should I drink with the medicine?

○ How long does it take the medicine to start working (called "onset of action")?

○ Is it safe to drink alcoholic beverages, drive, or operate machinery after I have taken pain medicine?

○ What side effects from the medicine are possible and how can I prevent them?

You won't become addicted

When I had the worst pain from my epididymitis, I was furious at the doctors who were giving me aspirin and other ineffective antiinflammatories, and who didn't seem to care that I was in pain. As my life seemed to deteriorate, and I found it impossible to work and carry on human communication without constantly complaining or feeling out of it (way out of it), I did keep asking around. Finally, I found a pain clinic at Beth Israel Hospital in New York City. The specialist I saw could tell immediately that I was in a lot of pain, and that something had to be done. She was amazed that no one had given me Percocet or anything "that simple" to see if it would work. By then, I knew that many doctors are afraid to become involved with self-administered opioids, but this woman had no such fear. She put a nurse in the room with me, gave me a single Percocet tablet and told me to stay there for an hour. They wanted to make sure I had no adverse reactions.

On the contrary, within a few minutes—maybe ten—I could feel a tiny bubble (I use the term descriptively, not as a real thing) forming in my body. Within twenty minutes, the pain I'd had for six months was gone!

I left there with a prescription for a bottle of the medicine, instructions to take four to eight tablets a day, and to call if the pain got worse. Over the next four days, I took only four pills in total, breaking them in half and stretching out the dosage. I was afraid of addiction, even if my doctor wasn't. Within the week, my pain was gone, and didn't come back for over a year. I stopped taking the medicine after those four days, and have used it only when the pain comes back. I've also used it for back pain and tendinitis—sparingly.

This may sound like a miraculous recovery, but it is similar to many stories I hear all the time. Pain control is possible, and simply has to be explored, a day at a time.

Any cautions?

When used properly, these medications are safe, but don't abuse them. Don't take more than you're told to take. Don't get prescriptions from more than one physician and pile them on top of each other.

If you get what's called "breakthrough pain" (pain that suddenly comes out of nowhere after most has been under control), don't hesitate to take another tablet. Keeping pain under control requires keeping ahead of the curve. But if you find yourself doing that often, discuss the matter with your doctor, as he might need to adjust the dosage or change your medication entirely if it has stopped being effective for you.

Finally, don't compare your pain medication and control to someone's else. All patients are different. Pain is different for each individual. Different medications and different doses work in a variety of ways for you than for others.

Medications other than opioids

Surprisingly, many kinds of medications other than opioids may have a positive effect on your pain. A short list includes:

○ Some antidepressants
○ Some antihistamines
○ Some antianxiety drugs
○ Some amphetamines
○ Some steroids

Naturally, none of these should be taken without consulting a physician and getting a prescription. Never "borrow" drugs from a friend to see if they "work." And that goes double if you are already taking other medications at the same time, especially opioids, as the combination may cause unpleasant or even dangerous interactions. Codeine, for example, can intensify the effects of other drugs in your system, in ways that resemble an overdose. (Using the same pharmacy for all your prescriptions is another safeguard against mixing medications; most computerize their prescription information and will question a request that could create an unwanted interaction.)

One final note about opioids

Family or friends may give you all sorts of stories about what will happen to you if you "go down the road" of taking opioids for your pain.

Most of these will be myths that bear little or no relation to reality.

The field of pain control and palliative care have come a long way in the past five years.

There is a lot more known about what happens to people when they are in pain and take drugs, as compared to those who take drugs for the high.

People who take pain medications relax and feel better able to cope with the world. People who take the same drugs for highs are less able to cope.

One important myth to put down is that you will become desensitized to your pain medication, and therefore have to take more and more until it never works, or until you become addicted to it.

This is just not true. First of all, many people never become desensitized. What may happen is that the underlying cancer is causing greater pain, and that this increase in pain requires you to take more of your medication. Second, even if you become somewhat inured to the effects of the opioids, it is highly unlikely that you will become addicted.

All that will be required, should your condition ameliorate so that these drugs are no longer needed, is that you will gradually taper off your use of them. (Again, check with your doctor; going completely cold turkey from a full dosage regimen could shock your system.)

IN A SENTENCE:

> *There are many ways to control pain, including new palliative treatments—there is no reason for you to live in pain.*

living

It's OK to Lighten Up

IN MY wife Susan's first novel, *Fat Emily*, one of the characters is irked when the heroine of the book cracks a joke during a crisis. Her lover says, "Can't you ever be serious?" She counters, "This is too important to be serious."

I wish I could say that I've faced every challenge with a sense of humor. I wish I could say that I've kept up with Susan's dry, wise wit that undercuts people who are too pompous for their own good. She used to have a test for college boys on first dates. She'd ask them to take her to see Lenny Bruce. If the experience was too much for them, then she knew they weren't right for her. Well, if there was anything Lenny would understand, it's cancer!

When I was in the hospital for that operation on my abdomen, the recovery period was very long. They had removed a small, noncancerous tumor but I continued to be worried that it might precede other discoveries—of more developed cancer. It turns out I was wrong, but at the time I was depressed and anxious. The pain from my incisions, small as they were, was also upsetting. As I walked 'round and 'round the hospital floor—in a ritual ordered by the nursing staff every day to exercise my hurting muscles and increase my strength—I cursed the doctors who had put me through all this. Were it not for visits from my family, the six days spent in the hospital after the operation would have been totally miserable.

But there was something else that happened that taught me a big lesson in recovery. A little notice got posted at the door to the arts and crafts room on my floor (a room noticeable by the absence of anyone doing anything most of the time). It announced the performance on Sunday of a group called the Hamptons Comedy Festival.

As a press release on the Internet put it,

> The HCF was founded by television producer Abby Russell, who saw first-hand how comedy heals when her father recovered from prostate cancer. The first annual Hamptons Comedy Festival in 2000, second annual Hamptons Comedy Festival in 2001 and the third annual Hamptons Comedy Festival in 2002 earned public and industry kudos. The Festival garnered nods from many print, radio, and TV outlets, such as *Time Out New York* magazine, *New York* magazine, WOR Radio, and BBC Television in London.

Great, I thought, they want me to laugh my stitches out. I remembered all too well that childhood joke that ends with a punch line of "It hurts only when I laugh." If that sounds a little curmudgeonly, it's not surprising. I had had a scare, I had been in pain, and I wanted out of the hospital.

Two days later, however, I sat and laughed until it hurt (literally) and enjoyed it! For one hour, I actually forgot about cancer and pain and what might happen, as I listened to good comedians do good humor. Whether laughing can actually make your cancer go away—as some have suggested—is too controversial for me even to address. But I can assert with certainty, and from my own experience, that laughing can make you feel better emotionally, and can make you feel healthy. In other words, laughter is good medicine.

While writing a book on how to live with chronic illness, I later found there was a study at the Jonsson Cancer Center at the University of California–Los Angeles (UCLA), looking into the effects of laughter on the immune system of ill children and adolescents. This had never been done before, certainly not in the careful double-blind fashion that Jonsson was doing it.

A financial grant from the cable network, Comedy Central, is being used at Jonsson, says Larry Divney, president and chief executive officer of Comedy Central, to heighten people's awareness of the benefits of laughter.

"We know our programming is entertaining, but to think that I may discover that comedy is literally good for you is a very exciting proposition," he said.

One of the researchers was quoted as saying, "If you make people laugh, they don't get as anxious and they deal better with pain and do better in the hospital." (For more about the Jonsson study and Comedy Central's role, look in the Resource section at the end of this book.)

Of course, you don't have to watch Comedy Central to inject some humor into your life.

Many people with serious illnesses have found that by reading light literature, watching comedy DVDs, and telling stupid jokes to family members, they can lighten their burden.

Spouses, children, friends of someone who has cancer are likely to tip-toe around the patient, worried about upsetting him. They may think that acting silly or telling jokes or taking in a fun video together is somehow disrespectful to the seriousness of the disease. They may discourage you from enjoying yourself because they interpret this as denial of or even harmful to your condition. And when this happens, those who actually have the cancer often think, "My God, if everyone is pussy-footing around me, maybe I'm sicker than I thought." If you're simply ill, looking forward to many more years of life, hand in hand with watchful waiting or treatment, but everyone around you acts as if you are dying, it can be downright depressing.

My children made it a rule to keep me laughing. When I got lymphoma fifteen years ago, and there was some fear I might have to undergo chemotherapy for it, my youngest said, "Oh, Dad, don't let them do that. It'll make your hair fall out." Since I'm bald now, it was clearly a joke. A bad one. A stupid one. But, nonetheless, a joke. And I needed a joke at that point in time! So, I laughed. We all laughed. And it was a relief.

After that, I decided that laughter, stupid jokes, and bad comedy might not be a terrible way of getting through the period of treatment. I found that watching the reruns of *Whose Line is it Anyway?* was a wonderful way to spend an hour or two.

Later, as the periodic tests and announcements of remission kept coming up, I leveled the playing field a little bit by planning a vacation either just before or just after my six-month visits to the oncologist (with its depressing repetition of CAT scans, X-rays, blood tests, etc.).

By the time my prostate cancer came along, I knew some of the tricks. I scheduled my evenings around bad comedy shows. I told puns at work. And I made sure I had people around me who liked laughter and vacations.

All play a role in making recovery easier emotionally, whether they have anything to do with making it easier physically or not. And what—just for the sake of speculation—if they *did* have a positive effect on your physical health? Wouldn't that be a grand added bonus!

But how can a person have fun at a time like this?

There are people who are so debilitated emotionally by cancer that they cannot contemplate enjoying themselves. This is not because their physical condition prohibits it. Certainly, with prostate cancer, it is the rare case that your health will be so harmed you'll be unable to take a vacation. But your anxiety about your future might make you depressed. All the more reason why you would benefit from laughter.

But all the more reason why you might find it difficult to enjoy yourself.

This is another place where counseling can help. But, for the sake of humoring me, try this: after supper, go to your TV and turn to the worst sitcom you can find—something truly ridiculous. See if just watching this junk doesn't, in some way, distract you from your misery. And if this does it, then how about some recently released film everyone is talking about—whichever one "sets them howling" in the aisles? Or, check out vintage comedy films or even what had been your favorite cartoons when you were a kid. You enjoyed them then, you may well do so with renewed pleasure now. Even a little gallows humor might hit the spot—most public libraries have in their collection books featuring the cartoons of Charles Addams or Gahan Wilson, for instance.

I'm not trying to diminish the negative emotional effect on you of a diagnosis. I'm not trying to demean you by saying that when you're depressed you have to compound it by doing something beneath your dignity to try to cheer yourself up. I know how awful it is to be diagnosed, to have cancer. But I am saying that even in the depths of your fear and mental pain, it's possible to laugh; and that laughing, in and of itself, can have wonderful healing qualities.

IN A SENTENCE:

> *Laughter need not be a guilty pleasure at a time like this.*

You Are Not Cancer, You *Have* Cancer

learning

She sits straight up in her chair, a charming woman in her midfifties, thick glasses somewhat hiding her sharp blue eyes, diminishing the energy that her voice and demeanor express. She answers my questions unhesitatingly, talking about her metastasized breast cancer with honesty and strength.

"I don't want to be a patient. I want to be a person—right up until the end."

And she did so, continuing to go to work, to interact with her family, to carry on daily details, until—two years later—the disease took over her entire body and, at the age of fifty-eight, she died, surrounded by hospice workers and friends.

LUCKILY, FEW of you will ever face this woman's predicament. You will not become this ill; you will not die of painful, metastasized cancer. Prostate cancer is not breast or kidney or spleen cancer. It is, as I have said throughout this book, the slow-growing cancer that more men get than any other, but that few die of.

But, and this might surprise you, many men scare themselves *thinking* about how bad it could get. Many will find themselves living the life of a "cancer patient," not that of a functioning *person*.

What I want to do here is to sort out some of these thoughts and put them into perspective.

There are two conflicting points of view that a man could have. One is that you will never be the same again, that a diagnosis of cancer changes one's life forever. The second is that you are exactly who you were before, that nothing has changed about you except the diagnosis. The truth is somewhere in between.

Who you will never be again

> I woke the other day, and thought, "My God, I've got cancer. How long will I be with my children? How long will I be able to work?'

> My wife was crying, and I asked her what the matter was. "Nothing," she said. But I knew what it was: I was no longer immortal. I was a cancer victim.

> I used to be a carefree guy—going where I wanted, doing what I wanted. I play golf. I go to the office, work long hours. I love it. Now, I'm more afraid. I don't like it!

We are working, loving beings. No matter what we are inside, no matter how we try to talk ourselves into a different view of ourselves, our culture has determined that work and love are the crucial definers of manhood. Can we go on working, bringing in the money to sustain our family? Can we go on loving, having sexual pleasure and giving sexual pleasure? These two questions can be answered in the negative or the affirmative. Prostate cancer makes us think the only answer is the former.

I personally had planned to be with my wife until I was ninety-five. We used to joke about it. Both of us, in "the home," or in rocking chairs on our front porch. I wanted to see my great-grandchildren graduate college. Once I got prostate cancer, I wasn't sure any of that would happen.

"I don't know." That's a statement that any of us could make about our future at any point in our lives. But how much more poignant it is when you're thinking about cancer, when you're wondering if you'll ever get to do the traveling and loving and grandparenting you always planned.

"Who am I?" That's another question all of us pose at various times in our life. While a teenager: "Do people like me?" Later: "Am I a good potential husband? Am I a good person? Am I a good parent?" We like to believe we can control some of these attributes, that we can change our personality or, at least, our behavior to make us better friends or lovers or parents or citizens. Illness or disease—especially cancer—can rob us of this sense of control. We now see ourselves as patients: we are sick; we are somehow diminished or weak in character and, perhaps, in body.

Life stories

One of the ways that people who are coming to the end of their life can deal with the spiritual and psychological angst is to look back and tell their life story to someone. It's amazing what happens: they find out how many accomplishments they've been responsible for, how much love they've given and received. It turns out to be a very fulfilling and releasing experience. Because, at such times, focused so tightly on looking ahead, people often forget how much they've done and who they've been.

You're not at the end of your life; you're not dying. But the Life Story concept can be useful to you, too:

○ When have you been ill before? How did it turn out?
○ What about loved ones? How did you deal with their illnesses?
○ What goals did you have that you achieved? What goals are yet to be achieved?
○ Think of all the good times you've had. Think of the bad times.
○ What work has given you the most pleasure? What the least?
○ Whom have you loved? From whom have you wanted more love?

By looking backward, by charting the course of your previous life experiences, you can put your present circumstances more into perspective. By seeing how much you've accomplished or gotten through, you can alleviate some of your anxiety about the future. By seeing how much you've loved and been loved, you may appreciate those close to you with renewed thankfulness.

When Joseph Santiago first got married, he and his wife were only nineteen. They had no family to support them, no college education. They had to take whatever jobs they could. Along about the third year of their marriage, Maria Santiago asked where they were going to take their vacation that year. "We can't afford one," Joseph said. "We can't afford *not* to take one," his wife answered.

For the thirty years of their marriage, with three children growing up, then in college, and now out of the house, the Santiagos *did* take a yearly vacation. Now, having been diagnosed with prostate cancer, Joseph can look back on the wonderful experiences he would never have had were it not for his wife's insistence.

Today

Looking back, perhaps you see things you'd done or said or thought that you wish you hadn't. Perhaps there are things you haven't done that you wish you had.

Diagnosis with an illness can sharpen a perception of who you are today, and who you would like to be. It can make you think about what your life goals were, and what they *could* yet be. This awareness may be your opportunity to shape your present circumstances to what you will be happy to look back on, without regrets.

There may be activities and people whom you have long wished—or only now realize—you can drop from your life. Doing so may be an enormous relief. Reevaluating what is truly important to you can make you think of giving up some of the drudgery of life, in favor of taking on more of its pleasures. As the saying goes, you only live once.

After my diagnosis of lymphoma and prostate cancer, though I was still relatively young (in my early sixties), I realized that I was working harder than I really wanted to. I needed the income, but maybe I could slip in some other activities that I enjoyed. I began to take piano lessons, and joined a local Shakespeare production company. I took acting lessons.

Yes, you may still wake in the morning and say to yourself, "Even if I am not going to die of this, I now know I will die someday of something." Yes, if your treatment has caused impotence, you may have to admit to yourself, "I can't be the lover I once was." And, yes, these are painful redefinitions of self. But look beyond the illness. What has bugged you for many years that now seems—and can *be*—less important because it's seen in the light of your cancer? What suddenly feels really important to do, or become?

Think of this time as a kind of New Year's Day, when you can make resolutions that you will *keep*. What has seemed an arduous or onerous task may now feel easier, next to the enormity of what you have just been through. Think of the books you want to read, the people you want to meet, the traveling you want to do, a second career you've always made some excuse not to pursue. While this tap on your shoulder is *only that*—it is not a death knell—nonetheless it is a wakeup call, a second chance to decide how to make the best use of the rest of your life.

When someone asks how you feel, when you go back for checkups, when your anxiety kicks in, remind yourself that it's *only* prostate cancer, not something more serious, but that you can make your life more interesting, better, more exciting, less painful if you use this experience to appreciate the bounty and possibilities of your present life, expel from it what you don't want and plan for the future.

Who you may become and still are—the future

As my father-in-law used to say, "*J* stands for *Just a Minute!*"

There is nothing about prostate cancer that really changes who you are. You are still the head of your family, still the good parent, still the valued employee, still handsome or funny or jovial or ugly or depressed. Cancer isn't the determinant: your *view* of cancer is the determinant of how you react to what you're going through.

A person's personality and character will usually not (some people will say it *cannot*) change because of a diagnosis of prostate cancer. Your life experience is just as valuable as it once was. However, how you *use* that experience may change if you react to this disease in an inappropriate way, one that assumes you've changed. But *you haven't* changed. Your body may do things a little differently, you may have some anxieties that you never had before, but overall you are still who you were before this diagnosis and treatment. Your values and your intellectual capabilities remain.

Still, your goals can be reevaluated. Envision who you will be, five years from now and cancer-free. What will be your work, if you will be working? Who will matter most to you personally? What will occupy your spare time and thoughts? What good things to come out of your present experience do you see yourself continuing, such as exercising or eating better, going for checkups even when nothing is wrong, taking time out to enjoy yourself more?

My Shakespeare, Joseph Santiago's new appreciation of vacations: these could be yours if the diagnosis of cancer knocks you about a bit and puts you in a different frame of mind. Some of this takes planning, but you can do that now, as you are on the path to feeling and becoming well. This is the perfect time to work with friends or colleagues or your wife on ways you'd like to change your present lifestyle, from family activities or trips to new personal pursuits or even a different kind of work. And, to communicate to those you care for, how much they mean to you.

If you can use cancer as the excuse to finally get rid of that potbelly that's been bothering you for fifteen years; if you can say "I love you" to your friends and family at least once a day; if you can say, "Thank God, it's *only* prostate cancer;" if you can start a *new* relationship with someone whom you've always admired; if you can do something that will make you admire *yourself* more—then this entire experience, including the fright it has given you, may change your life for the better. Not just your future, but how you now view your entire life.

One more example from my own life: I have always known that life was not endless. In fact, for many of the middle years of my life, I would worry about every cut finger, every cough, every pain in my body, thinking that it meant some serious illness that might end my life prematurely. I was not quite a hypochondriac, but I was worried about adverse symptoms and what they might portend. Would I live even to be sixty, sixty-five, seventy?

Now that I'm past 70, with lymphoma and prostate cancer tucked away into the past, I find that I no longer worry about longevity. Each day, each year, is a bonanza. I feel better, I do more, I even *think* better. I'm working at a full-time job, I'm writing, I'm playing the piano, I'm acting in plays, and I'm waiting for my first grandchild and my next vacation.

To some extent, it was my experience with *cancer* that gave me that perspective.

IN A SENTENCE:

> *Now is the time to appreciate and build upon all those facets of your life untouched by cancer.*

living

What If It Comes Back?

I WANT to tell you a little story about my own anxiety during both my bouts with lymphoma and prostate cancer. It comes from a diary I kept some twelve years ago.

It is June 2, and I am standing in the middle of a dusty street in the one-horse town of Pecos, New Mexico. Across the road is the Pecos Trading Company, where hand-tooled leather saddles sit side by side with Stetson hats and old phonograph records, struggling to catch the tourist's eye. Wildflowers dot the verge, cattle wander in the distance, and the faraway mesas attest to ancient peoples and an ancient geology.

Susan and I have gone away for a week, partly because we're due a vacation, partly to celebrate the passing of one full year in the saga of my lymphoma. Memorial Day 1992 was the key point in discovery; Memorial Day 1993 has come and (just) gone and I am still alive.

Now, however, in the middle of this quiet, venerable land, down the road from one of the oldest settlements in North America, where ancient native cultures clashed with the Spanish invaders, I am talking on the only pay phone in town—long distance to the hospital in New York, trying to reach Dr. B. The reason is that I have awakened in the middle of the night to discover that one of my clavicle bones—the right side, where all the radiation was concentrated—is swollen and painful. My mind leaps: shall I tell Susan? Is it an aberration of the dust and heat of the Southwest, or is this a wild and damaged cell, screaming that it needs attention? Or is it something else—something equally benign or equally malignant? Bone cancer, perhaps. The imagination of the fearful is unlimited.

I do tell Susan and, together, out there in the dusty streets of Pecos, New Mexico, we hang onto the phone, trying to reach my doctors.

"Tender is better," Dr. B. tells me, when the operator finally understands the panic in my calls and connects me to him. "Lymphomas are generally not tender or sore." Fine, but what about bone cancer or radiation poisoning or . . . ? The mind wanders on, plotting dangers and disasters. Susan and I are victims of fear, and we realize that I may be healthy for many years to come, but the pinpoint of cold terror will still rise up in us at a moment's notice, transforming us into cowering beasts or primitive humans. It is a contradiction of our humanity that we cannot—at this point in time—change and accept the possibility that nothing is wrong.

That it all turns out to be nothing more than a torn muscle from whitewater rafting the day before makes no difference in our psyches. Within our brains, we know that I've been lucky, that I'm not seriously ill, that lymphoma is a treatable disease.

What I wrote about lymphoma could also hold true for prostate cancer. I offer you my experience only so that you can know that at least one other person in the universe has felt that shiver of unnatural anxiety about the future after supposedly successful treatment for cancer.

Is it a cure or remission?

Your chances of being alive, and disease-free, five or ten years after diagnosis are apt to depend more on the stage and grade of your cancer than on your choice of treatment.[1] One of the problems—as well as the benefits—of having this cancer as contrasted with many others, is that remission can be very long; so long that you won't be able to distinguish between remission and cure. After all, what is cure? It's the idea that you won't ever have the disease again in such a fashion that it (a) needs treatment; (b) causes you pain; or (c) kills you. A long, long remission, one that ends in your death at an advanced age from something other than prostate cancer, seems to me to be as good as a cure.

That having been said, you will still want to know your chances of staying relatively disease-free for the rest of your life. You will want to know whether your treatment has "worked." You will want to die a natural death at an advanced age. You don't want to spend all those years living in fear of metastases.

The best I can tell you is what the experts tell me: If you are above the age of sixty-five and have started out with a slow-growing tumor with well-differentiated cells, then you have a very good chance, according to the latest knowledge, of not having to worry about prostate cancer again. Which is why my doctor asked if I wanted to be "cured" and said that the radiation would do that. (Nonetheless, he does still want me to see him once a year, just to check everything is OK.)

The NCI reports that a survey of prostate cancer patients showed that,

> Ten years after a prostatectomy for localized cancer, prostate cancer had claimed the lives of 6 percent of the men whose cancers were well-differentiated compared with 20 percent of those with moderately differentiated cancers and 23 percent of those with poorly differentiated cancers. The chances of developing metastatic prostate cancer followed a similar pattern.
>
> Ten years after surgery, metastases had been diagnosed in 13 percent of the men with well-differentiated tumors, but in 32 percent of those with cancers that were moderately differentiated and 48 percent of those whose cancers were poorly differentiated.

Those double-digit figures must seem very frightening, contradicting what I just said. What you have to realize is that, in statistical medical terms, a 13 percent metastases rate for well-differentiated tumors is a good rate. You also have to take these numbers with some salt. This is only one survey. You don't know the population, and you don't know what has been done since that survey to upgrade chances of remission.

Let me give you another survey, this one taken from looking at the outcomes from many different sources.

This analysis showed survival of ten years for 94 percent of men with Gleason scores as high as 4, 75 percent survival of ten years for Gleasons up to 7.[2]

As usual, with this disease, you ask a question and you get several, often disparate answers.

Higher Gleasons

The bad news is that there is no real way of determining whether a slow-growing tumor may turn into an aggressive one; no way of curing an aggressive metastatic one.

The hope for those small number of men with very aggressive, already metastasized tumors is threefold:

- ○ Hormone therapy
- ○ Palliation for pain and other symptoms
- ○ New treatments already in the pipeline (see Learning)

The message is clear. None of us is home free.

On the other hand, being anxious a lot of the time about "what ifs" is not useful. For most of us, we have a reasonably good chance that we're home free. So live as much as you can with the attitude that you are in that lucky majority.

IN A SENTENCE:

> *There is good evidence that, treated or not, many men will survive ten to fifteen years after diagnosis.*

learning

New Treatments on the Horizon

RESEARCH IS not as revolutionary or cutting-edge as one might wish. In fact, most of what's "new" in research for prevention and treatment, consists of honing and combining tools already in use, as well as getting more precise about what the numbers mean when a PSA or biopsy is completed.

Is anything truly new?

That said, it doesn't mean that there is no cutting-edge research out there. The NCI and the National Institutes of Health (NIH) list the following as current research efforts:[3]

○ Scientists are exploring new treatment schedules and ways of combining various types of treatment, such as radiation therapy and hormonal therapy.
○ They are studying the effectiveness of chemotherapy to kill cancer cells.
○ They are studying biological therapy—using the body's immune system.
○ Researchers are also studying drugs to lessen the side effects of treatment, such as bone loss.

○ Surgeons at some medical centers are exploring the use of laparo-scopic prostatectomy. The surgeon makes several tiny incisions rather than a single long incision.

○ For men with early-stage prostate cancer, researchers are comparing immediate treatment with surgery (or radiation) against watchful waiting. This study delays giving treatment to men in the watchful-waiting group until they have symptoms. The results of the study will help doctors know whether to treat early stage prostate cancer immediately or only later on, if symptoms occur or get worse.

Here are some other things that scientists are working on:

○ In December 2004, there was a report that green tea can be a factor in the prevention of prostate cancer. To be more precise, within green tea are **polyphenols**, which apparently keep malignant prostate can-cer cells from growing and spreading. Since green tea has long been given by alternative medicine groups and advocates as a beneficial drink for a wide variety of ailments, including various cancers, it is good to get some bona fide scientific evidence that this is so.

○ A really big piece of news came out in the summer of 2003: the first truly effective drug to prevent prostate cancer. It turns out that a long-term study on a drug called finasteride—which affects hormone levels in men—showed a decided decrease in the development of prostate cancer as against men who took only a placebo (the study involved nine thousand men). The downside of this study was that the men who did develop cancer during the study appeared to develop more high-grade, virulent cancer, the kind that spreads. However, further study of these men is necessary to see if they do indeed develop more advanced cancer. It's important to note that nothing in the report about this drug trial indicated that finasteride was any help for people who had already developed prostate cancer. In terms of side effects, incontinence was not a problem; however, impotence was slightly increased.[4]

○ Hormone therapy has long been a treatment given to men either before or after surgery or radiation. The protocol has been three years of **androgen**-reducing hormone treatment, given because it (a) reduces tumors prior to surgery; and (b) has a beneficial effect on long-term return or growth of the cancer. Now, scientists at Boston's Brigham and Women's Hospital and Dana-Farber Cancer Institute report in the *Journal of the American Medical Association* that only six months of such treatment seems to have a more helpful effect on men treated with radiation than men who had radiation alone. Four important notes about this study: (a) It was done on men who had cancer only within their prostate; (b) the cancer studied was of a low stage, but one that eventually becomes aggressive; (c) long-term hormone treatments have harmful side effects, so the shorter term is considered an important benefit; and (d) not enough work has been reported to make this the norm for treatment, yet.[5]

○ There is, for the first time, a little evidence that some combinations of chemotherapy might extend life a couple of months for men whose hormone therapy is no longer reducing pain and tumor growth in advanced prostate cancer that has spread. The importance here, obviously, is that this might mean that eventually some chemotherapy will be useful to treat larger groups of men—and extend life longer.[6]

○ Another study takes advantage of developments in understanding the workings of DNA and the human genes. Which mutations in genes might mean some men will develop prostate cancer and which don't? To do this study, scientists are looking mainly at families in which the disease has cropped up in a number of individuals. "Stay tuned," as they say.[7]

○ As reported in Month Four, the effect of vitamins and other supplements to your diet are being studied in several clinical trials. Can lycopene and other tomato products actually prevent or slow down prostate cancer? Again, it's way too early for definitive news.[8]

○ Diets high in veggies and fruits but low in fat are being examined to see if they really can make a difference in who does or does not develop prostate cancer, especially a return of the disease.

○ More and more researchers are applying for grants to check out more radical ways of treating prostate cancer, whether it be through freezing, biological, or chemical breakthroughs. For instance, at the University of Michigan, the Urologic Oncology Program received a grant of $5.7 million for what the NCI calls a Specialized Program of Research Excellence (SPORE) grant.

○ Active laboratory programs include work in the areas of great interest, including "prostate cancer genetics, gene discovery, prostate cancer metastasis, prostate immunology, prostate carcinogenesis, and
prostate and bladder cell biology."

○ Interestingly, they're also looking at quality-of-life issues as having
an affect on the disease after and during treatment for prostate
cancer that has metastasized.

○ A group of physicians from Idaho, calling themselves CancerConsultants (they have a Web site, http://patient.cancerconsults.com)
have issued a paper, authored by Charles H. Weaver, MD, managing editor of CancerConsultants, and C. D. Buckner, MD, the
group's scientific editor, in which they talk in great detail about the
use of new hormone treatments, given trials in England, that can
have a substantive positive effect both on quality of life and slowing
of growth if given to men who are not symptomatic.

○ On the negative front, there is now clear evidence that, for a very
small group of men who use it, the pesticide methyl bromide gas can
be one cause of prostate cancer. This is a group of individuals who
are professionally engaged in pest control and spray the gas in large
doses over a long period of time.[9]

For more descriptions of some of the work being done abroad you might
turn to Month Eleven's Learning section.

IN A SENTENCE:

> *There are numerous, fascinating studies concerning new treat-
> ments for and the prevention of prostate cancer.*

living

Depression and Anger

> I began to sleep a lot more than usual. And I wasn't interested in playing the piano anymore. When I went to my oncologist, he said that it probably wasn't due to the treatments. So I went to my internist. She ran all sorts of tests: thyroid, blood, urine—all the regular stuff. Nothing came out. She said I was really healthy, despite my cancer. She suggested I could just be depressed. Depressed! I'd never been depressed in my life.—FRANK

FRANK'S EXPERIENCE is not unusual at all. What's unfortunate is that the oncologist didn't warn Frank about the possibility of depression, and didn't recognize the symptoms when they came up.

The fact is, anywhere from three months to nine months, as you're getting over the physical effects of your treatment (later, if you had surgery; sooner if it was radiation), emotional reactions begin to set in.

Is what you are feeling depression?

Sure, you've had emotional ups and downs before this. Perhaps you were anxious waiting to hear how bad the cancer was, where it had spread (if anywhere), and trying to decide what treatment to have. But this is different. You're apathetic, exhausted, out of sorts—signs of depression.

For those who don't necessarily know what it's like to be depressed, who think they're just tired or worried in the everyday sense, here's a list of symptoms that I find useful:

- ○ You're sure you've made terrible errors, but not quite sure where.
- ○ You think that anything that goes wrong is your fault.
- ○ You feel a heaviness in the chest and limbs.
- ○ You'd like to go to bed and sleep a lot more than you used to.
- ○ Sometimes, you even wish you were dead.
- ○ And, in the worst case, you actually try to end depression with suicide.

Millions of Americans have these symptoms for reasons other than cancer; many live with them for a long time without doing anything about them. Others get medication for **endemic** depression. It's true that depression has many causes, and some requires long-term psychotherapy as well as medication to get under control. But your depression probably comes from the very simple fact that you've been through a very frightening situation, one that often can lead to situational depression—a state of mind triggered by actual events rather than imagined ones.

You may have believed that, once the treatment was over, you'd feel better, emotionally as well as physically. Now, though, you're upset and may not understand why.

Where these feelings come from

Here's an analogy. When a child goes through a first separation from his or her parents—say, a sleepaway at a friend's—the youngster often has no emotional distress during the event. But when the child comes home, watch out! Then is when all the anxiety and anger about being "sent away" comes out. Parents often are baffled by tantrums after a pleasant experience like that ("Your daughter was a perfect angel," says the mother of the child's friend) but they are most likely the stored-up anxiety at a first-time experience. The thing is, you see, that it's now safe for the child to express her fears or anger. Maybe she was too young—or felt she was too young—to go away. Maybe she was simply experiencing those worries that children normally feel when they do something a little too daring, and then blame their parents for not stopping them.

Similarly, you may have gotten through your diagnosis and subsequent testing, and your choice to have treatment was your own, but perhaps you chose to bury your stronger feelings during these difficult months that have just passed. Now, when you are feeling safe, the anger and anxiety are surfacing. But maybe you don't think it's "right" to express anger or fear, so the result is depression.

This is a very common experience, in reaction to a very real, threatening event.

This isn't the only emotional reaction you may have at about this time. You could also experience anxiety that doesn't seem to be in response to anything real. In the middle of the night, the cold sweats come over you, the icy fingers of terror, the thumping of your heart in your chest. You may be afraid to travel—though you loved that trip to Africa just last year. You may be afraid that your daughter isn't making enough money at her new job, when you've never been worried about that kind of thing before. You've probably seen people like this—men and women who are frightened of something, but they don't quite know of what, so they attach the anxiety to everyday things.

All of this could be because you've been through an experience that has shaken you up more than you thought. Having cancer showed you that maybe you weren't as in control of your life as you'd thought you were, and now everything seems uncertain or effortful.

One of the ways that Frank discovered his depression was his sleepiness. But he also was surprised he didn't enjoy playing the piano. And one might guess that his wife found him irritable when she made suggestions about "getting out and enjoying yourself."

Depressed people just don't like having people tell them how to feel better.

The fact is, the emotional journey began with your diagnosis. It doesn't end when you've been treated and dealt with side effects. It's probably not going to stop until you have gone through several years of post-treatment checkups and, dare I say it, psychotherapy or counseling.

A lot of men reading this statement may resent my suggestion that they need therapy. But I cannot stress enough that the underlying emotions that go along with prostate cancer (not to mention any potentially life-threatening illness) are there even if you don't feel them. The mental health field is old enough and wise enough by now to be able to state with certainty that sad feelings that are not acknowledged—and dealt with—can have harmful effects on body and soul. Bottling them up does not make them go away.

Anger

Perhaps your feelings aren't bottled up—perhaps you are exploding. As I've suggested earlier in this chapter, anger is often the flip side of depression. It slips out when the depression itself becomes too burdensome, or when someone challenges your "downbeat mood." I, myself, have thundered things like, "Of course I'm downbeat. What the hell would *you* be if you had cancer!" Then, ashamed of my outburst, I return to the depressed state whence I came.

But anger can exist on its own, without depression. On one level, it's a perfectly natural and respectable response to danger. You may already have experienced that kind of reaction on being informed that you had cancer in the first place, or in anticipation of treatment.

Anger can, in fact, be the result of many kinds of circumstances and, as everyone knows, can be perfectly justified. What is harder to pinpoint, however, is anger that is *unjustified* when weighed against the immediate circumstances that are inspiring you to express it.

Anger at your doctor

After treatment, when your oncologist has told you that the cancer is taken care of, you may find yourself getting angry. But why? You're cured. (Answer: Up until now, you may have been afraid your emotions would overwhelm you. Now, you can let your emotional guard down.)

I know that *I* get angry every time I go to get a checkup. "What are those dummies doing?" I fret. "Why are they taking so long? Why are they spending so little time with me? Why don't they see me first? Why don't they apologize for . . . ?" On and on I go, forgetting that what I am really feeling (and this occurs year after year after year) is *anxiety* that the doctors may find something new; something dangerous. It's anxiety I am turning into anger. I want to shoot the messenger, even if all he has to bear is good news.

Other examples of anger

When someone asks you how you're doing, you may be irritable, annoyed by what may seem like prying rather than concern, or prodded into remembering that you have a disease you'd like to forget about once in a while.

You may snap at people when confronted by circumstances where you wouldn't have done so in the past. Everything from impatience with having to stand in line to road rage may be unusual to your character, and yet you find yourself with a hairline-trigger temper now.

You may simply be on edge generally, finding that any little thing gets on your nerves. This anger may be getting in the way of your being able to enjoy anything that you used to.

Anger is about control

Consider the following: perhaps you're one of those men who has not previously considered that life can run away from you; that events can affect you without your permission. Perhaps because you so pride yourself on controlling your world, you are both angered and frightened by an inability to do so. You hate having cancer because it makes you feel weak and ineffectual. You hate not being able to will it or pay it or punch it away.

Or perhaps you followed every health regimen you could, and now despite all your efforts, this cancer had to happen to you. Certainly it *is* frustrating and frightening to learn that your body is betraying you.

Anger, in the form of your having a strong effect upon who and what is nearest you, and perhaps even against your own body, is a way of demonstrating that maybe you really are back in control after all. But if what you are doing and saying is not what a situation really calls for, if the anger itself is ineffectual, you're really spinning out of control. You need to find a safe outlet for your feelings, something that won't damage those who matter to you.

Coping with anger

First, be aware that feelings of helplessness and of your body's betrayal may be behind your anger, if that anger is coming out at surprising moments that hitherto did not evoke such a strong reaction from you.

Second, as I've said several times elsewhere in this book, there's nothing wrong in seeking counseling to help you understand your anger and decrease it. You may not do this unless you personally find the outbursts unpleasant, or a loved one confronts you about your behavior, but just *knowing* that anger is a result of threats to one's sense of unity and control may help you curb an instinct to lash out.

On one level, anger is more healthy than depression, in that your feelings are more out in the open, but in the end it's not much fun for you and those close to you, is it? Once you recognize that anger may be a result of your diagnosis or treatment, you've taken the first step toward relieving it. Many of the solutions for depression would apply here, as would Month Eight's Living section on lightening up. You may also need to give yourself permission to grieve for your illness.

A *sense of loss*

One of the unexpected parts of any such illness—and particularly one in which your genitals are involved—is a sense of loss. A very smart dictum of the world of social work is that "all losses are the same." By this is not meant that the loss of a loved one is literally the same as the loss of a wallet; or that the loss of a limb is the same as the loss of sexual capability.

But there is a sameness as far as the symbolism of loss goes. There is a metaphorical loss that superimposes itself on all losses. And, make no mistake about it, you have lost something important if a part of your body is taken away, not to mention if you experience a diminishment of your sex life.

The present loss may remind you of earlier losses or disappointments— big and small—and you may feel bereft, whether you are aware of it or not.

So, you may wish to go back to the same person with whom you spoke when you were trying to decide on treatment, some eight months ago.

Or you may wish to find a therapist who can dig a little deeper into your feelings. This is especially valuable when the depression taps into fears and anger you may not immediately recognize—anger at the fact that you have been robbed of the ease with which you had hoped to face your future; fear that you may not be able to have sex again, or that you may get another cancer, or that this one will return.

Spiritual support

In addition to any emotional and psychological counseling you may seek at this time, many people turn to spiritual support as well.

I don't mean you have to get down on your knees and pray—though you certainly might, if that gives you support. I don't even mean that you have to talk with a minister or rabbi.

There are other ways to get support that is not quite physical and not quite emotional—which is what most people mean by spiritual, anyway.

One of these is **yoga**. For centuries, this discipline has provided calm and relaxation to tens of thousands of people. Interest in it surged during the 1970s, and continues today. I myself find the time and concentration necessary to practice yoga too difficult. In addition, my body is one of those inflexible physiques that don't accommodate themselves well to the practice.

But Mike Milken, whose own cancer started him on both a personal healing search and support for huge research projects nationwide, found that a variety of so-called New Age techniques were both soothing and—at least in his view—physically healing. The story about him and cancer in *Fortune* magazine outlines some of his practices in this arena. Among them are certainly the use of yoga, but also of aromatherapy.

This turning to Eastern medical philosophies can be a turn-off to some men. But others, especially those who grew up during the 1960s, have come to see that "New Age" is really a pejorative comment about ancient ideas that have—for many people—proven effective in spiritually soothing troubled minds and troubled bodies.

Spiritual counselors

Just as some men may reject the notion of a psychological counselor ("What good can she do me? I've got cancer, not a mental disorder?"), they may reject a spiritual counselor. They may confuse spirituality with religion. And though over 65 percent of Americans say they are religious, and attend church or synagogue or mosque regularly, men often also reject any "need" for religious figures like priests or rabbis or imams to attend to their needs. But think of it this way: such figures, quite aside from their faith, are also revered as wise men (or women).

Here's what one Zen Buddhist master said to me when I asked what he would do if he were to attend the bedside of a person who was seriously ill: "I think the first thing I would do is to listen. Just listen. People who are very ill don't need to hear what I have to say; they need to talk."

You may have two reactions to that statement: (a) You're no longer seriously ill; (b) You may think that's what a psychotherapist or other mental health counselor is for—to listen to you talk. With regard to the first point, you may no longer believe consciously that you are seriously ill. Your prostate cancer may have been eradicated. But you are probably not fooling your unconscious mind. You have been tapped on the shoulder and told in no uncertain terms that you are mortal. And no one forgets that kind of warning, denial or not.

As for point B, there are all sorts of counseling, and all sorts of counselors. A spiritual counselor is there to listen to your worries about spiritual matters. What are they? Things such as:

- Is there an afterlife?
- Did I do anything to deserve this cancer? Is God punishing me?
- How can I do better for my community and my family?

These are questions you may want to ask of someone who has the ability, first, to listen to you, and then to discuss the spiritual ramifications of what has been bothering you.

It is highly unlikely that you will be satisfied by some pious statements on the part of a counselor whose faith you do not actively observe. But you may very well be happy to hear reflections of how other people have dealt with these kinds of very primal queries, that cut across all faiths; and how important it is to deal with the deep questions of life and death when you have faced and walked away from a serious illness.

IN A SENTENCE:

> *The only way to rid yourself of anger or depression is to let it out, among people who can help you feel safe.*

learning

Support Groups

SEVERAL TIMES in this book, I've suggested "support groups" as a logical place to go to obtain emotional help or information about prostate cancer.

Of course, many men don't want to go around talking about their "issues" with prostate cancer, either because they feel it's not manly to go complaining, or because they're embarrassed.

I hope by now you've gotten over the embarrassment. Since this is a disease that's shared by many men, there's nothing unmanly about having the cancer or about its treatments' side effects.

As to complaining, there's nothing more beneficial than to complain to those who truly understand your feelings and physical problems. So—you may want to look for a support group near you.

There are basically two kinds: one is the kind run by hospitals and other organizations, which have professional leaders and affiliations. These very often are broken down into groups for men who have had different kinds of treatment, with perhaps yet another group for wives or partners.

The second kind of support group is those run by private individuals who have started their own groups. These latter are called . . .

Self-help groups

About fifteen years ago, I wrote a book about what it's like to be left behind by suicide.[1] In the course of doing research, I discovered the large number of self-help support groups scattered around the country. A particularly helpful organization in this arena was the New Jersey Self-Help Clearing House. They pointed me in the direction of a couple of groups who let me sit in. This kind of self-help group, as contrasted with support groups in general, was usually run by those who were "survivors" of a family suicide.

Without a professional (social worker or psychologist) to channel the discussions in the group, many survivors found they could go where they needed and wanted to go. Many actually didn't trust psychology, because their loved one hadn't been "saved" by the profession.

Here's what the National Self-Help Clearinghouse has to say about what it and other self-help clearinghouses can do for you:

> The National Self-Help Clearinghouse is a not-for-profit organization that was founded in 1976 to facilitate access to self-help groups and increase the awareness of the importance of mutual support. The clearinghouse provides a number of services:
>
> ○ Assists human service agencies to integrate self-help principles and practices into their service delivery.
> ○ Conducts training activities for self-help group leaders and for professional facilitators of support groups.
> ○ Provides consultation to public agencies to promote their capabilities to encourage and sustain mutual support groups.
> ○ Carries out research activities, including research about the effectiveness of self-help, the character of the self-help process, and relationships with the formal caregiving systems.
> ○ Provides information about and referral to self-help support groups and regional self-help clearinghouses.
> ○ Conducts media outreach, provides speakers, and publishes manuals, training materials, monographs, and policy papers.[2]

Other kinds of support groups

There's nothing wrong with you and your friends who have had prostate cancer sitting down and sharing information with each other, but in this field it's often best to do the chatting with at least one medically experienced person leading the group.

Many men, therefore, want to discuss these issues with a group of people who have had the same problem, in the presence of a social worker, nurse, or physician.

I don't think I can do better in terms of describing the value of these groups than to quote what I found on the Internet at a site called AllRefer.

> Support groups consist of people who have come together to share the common experiences and problems unique to their disease or condition.
>
> Support groups are organized to deal with four main sources of stress: mental or physical illness, addictive or obsessive behavior, personal crisis or life changes, and caring for disabled family members.
>
> In addition to being a place to meet people who share a common bond, support groups also help members in other ways. Through newsletters and regular contact with other people in similar situations, members receive up-to-date information regarding their disability and treatments that are available. Along with this sharing comes understanding and a sense of belonging. Research confirms that the coming together of people in trouble serves to increase self esteem, decrease anxiety and depression, and raise levels of overall well-being.

How to find a support group

Information on support groups in your area can be found in a variety of ways. Handbooks of community resources, including support groups, are usually available in local libraries and hospitals. Major groups are often listed in the Yellow pages under "social service agencies."[3]

Under "Other Resources" at the back of this book, you'll find a number of places you can look for such support groups. But my strong recommendation is that you ask at the hospital where you're being treated. Memorial Sloan-Kettering, for instance, has a large Posttreatment Resource Center. It provides not only access to support discussion groups, but occasional seminars and lectures on all sorts of cancer-related pain management and other issues.

IN A SENTENCE:

> *Joining a support group may enable you not only to release and share your emotions but also to exchange valuable information.*

living

The African American and Prostate Cancer

IT IS heartening that attention is finally being paid to the seriously inflated rate of prostate cancer among African Americans.

What is disheartening is that the black male population of this country should have to suffer from that rate, which is 50 percent higher than for white men.

In fact, prostate cancer in the United States is higher among African Americans than any other group, according to the Congressional Black Caucus Foundation (CBCF).[1] It's not only that blacks get diagnosed with prostate cancer much more than whites; it's that black men die from the disease at a rate that is twice that of white men. According to the CBCF, "Five-year survival rates are lower for African American men (66.4 percent during 1983 to 1990) than for white men (81.3 percent during 1983 to 1990)."[2]

And this is true even when the fact that African-American men get diagnosed later than whites is factored into the picture.

What's especially unfortunate is that prostate cancer grows faster in black men than in other population groups.

Why are African Americans targeted by prostate cancer?

The causes behind this extreme racial divide have yet to be determined. There are hypotheses, however.

Genetics

Since almost all cancers have some genetic component, there is no reason to doubt that that is true of prostate cancer as well, suggests Dr. Isaac Powell, chief of urology at the Veterans Administration Hospital of Detroit. He goes on to add that since hormones play an important role in the rate of growth of prostate cancer, and since different ethnic populations have differences in their hormone production and control, hormonal factors probably are partly to blame for cancer-related differences along ethnic lines.

Some years back, the CBCF reports, researchers at the University of Southern California published a report "that the risk of developing prostate cancer is five times as high for African-American and Latino men who carry [a gene] mutation in comparison to men without it."[3]

While this research is promising, the CBCF article also deplores the small amount of money (less than 2 percent of the NCI's budget yearly) that goes toward studying people of color.

The genome project

In the last few years, great strides have been taken in understanding the exact gene(s) that play a role in specific traits and illnesses. The hope is that, eventually, gene modification will allow scientists to "retrofit" our bodies to be healthier.

The National Human Genome Research Institute and Howard University looked at this matter of high rates of prostate cancer in African-American men in what they called "The National Cooperative Study of Hereditary Prostate Cancer in African Americans." What they found was a specific gene associated with "increased risk of prostate cancer." This is significant enough that I want to quote at some length from their report:

Ever since 1992, when Johns Hopkins researchers first showed that some forms of prostate cancer could be inherited, scientists have intensely searched for specific genes that cause the disease. In 1996, NHGRI scientists, in collaboration with researchers at Johns Hopkins and in Sweden, studied 91 high-risk prostate cancer families and mapped the first hereditary susceptibility to prostate cancer to a region of chromosome 1 that they called the Hereditary Prostate Cancer 1 Region, or HPC1. Since then, these and other research teams have mapped prostate cancer suscepibly genes to two other parts of chromosome 1, as well as to chromosomes 17, 20, and X.[4]

Following up on this discovery, scientists continue to look at these genes in both whites and African Americans, to find how the mutation may account for the higher and lower rates of prostate cancer.

Dietary differences

At the risk of sounding biased, one cannot ignore the high-fat meals that are available in many low-income, black neighborhoods—the popularity of fast foods, fried foods, and animal products that of course contain animal fats. This is a demographic fact, not an assumption on my part. As Dr. Powell points out, "African Americans have a higher fat content in their diet than other populations."

Some years back, the NCI also tried to tease out the causal factors in the disparity between whites and blacks. They added "diet during adolescence" to the package of risks.

Treatment modalities

Scientists have wondered if the treatments that African Americans receive for their prostate cancer might be responsible for the higher death rate. Or whether the kind of prostate cancer is different in African Americans than in whites. But, so far, these two approaches have not turned up any clues. A study in Texas, comparing radiation treatment in both groups, did not show any difference in recurrence or "cure rate" between whites and blacks.[5]

However, it is glaringly obvious that low-income African Americans do not get the same level of health care as more affluent ones, or of whites in general. Later diagnosis, or the failure to make a correct diagnosis, the high cost of treatment or unavailability of top-of-the-line medical centers . . . all of these play a part in the mortality rate for blacks.

Which leaves us where?

The present state of affairs is that scientists continue to probe the ethnic issue, and continue to urge African Americans to be screened for prostate cancer (via regular visits to their doctors for PSA tests and DREs), taking into account the disparity between financial capability and health insurance, not to mention availability of specialists for people of color in this country.

If you are black, this means you need far more than men of other races to become your own health advocate, to research and demand the best treatment, even if perhaps this means using doctors other than your usual physician or traveling beyond your locale to the most up-to-the-minute labs or treatment centers. Don't settle for becoming another statistic.

IN A SENTENCE:

> *Prostate cancer discriminates along racial lines, for reasons yet undetermined; if you are black, demand the care you need— your life depends on it.*

learning

Prostate Cancer Beyond the United States

WHILE THE Food and Drug Administration may not approve certain drugs or treatment techniques in the United States, that doesn't mean that the rest of the world is following suit. Here are some of the things that I discovered about what's going on elsewhere.

Ultrasound

In France, at the Institute of Health and Medical Research in Paris, scientists have been experimenting with high-intensity focused ultrasound (HIFU) to eliminate cancerous cells in men with Stage I or II prostate cancer. A firm named EDAP has created a device called Ablatherm that is now licensed for use in the European Union, Great Britain, Russia, and South Korea. A firm called Focus Surgery, located in Indianapolis, has created a similar device, called Sonablate. Both devices can work for other cancers.

While the technique is still in clinical trials in America (at the Indiana University Cancer Center and at Case Western University), researchers and officials in France have concluded that it is sufficiently effective and safe to be used for treatment.

Here's how it works: A patient with low-stage (contained) prostate cancer lies on his right side (much like during a colonoscopy) and is sedated, so that he won't move during the moderately long treatment (about two to three hours.) In addition, he is given a spinal anesthetic to eliminate any chance of pain. A probe is placed in the rectum. This probe emits a beam of high-intensity convergent ultrasound. In the point where the ultrasounds are focused, the sudden and intense absorption of the ultrasound beam creates a sudden elevation of the temperature (from 85°C to 100°C), which destroys the cells located in the targeted zone. The targeted zone destroyed by each shot is oval-shaped and measures about 22 mm in height by 2 mm in diameter. Repeating the shots, and moving the focal point between each shot, it is possible to destroy a volume that includes the whole tumor.[6]

The reason to use HIFU rather than surgery or radiation is that it has as good a rate of getting rid of the cancer while halving the rate of impotence, and it also makes incontinence much less likely.[7] It works for those men who don't want or can't have surgery or radiation because of other medical problems or complications.

Also, HIFU seems to work for patients who have a recurrence of the cancer after radiation. And while a full course of radiation cannot be used more than once on any individual patient, the makers of Ablatherm and the Paris Institute say that HIFU can.

As with any treatment, follow-up visits, including biopsies, are recommended for some years, and there are some side effects. This is, after all, a medical procedure. A catheter for urine is used, and kept in for two to three days, and this can cause an infection. However, antibiotics treat that very handily. And the side effects are not anywhere near as certain or dangerous as those that may occur following surgery.

As of July 2004, five thousand men have been treated in Europe with HIFU, and the results—according to the manufacturer—are that 92 percent have had negative follow-up biopsies and stable PSA tests.

What does all this mean for American men? If you want to go to Europe to get this treatment, you can, though most American insurers (including Medicare) will not pay for it. You can also keep track of the progress of this treatment through the FDA and the NCI.

Gene therapy

In studies performed in the United Kingdom, the BBC reports that a specific gene (called IGF1R) may play a role in prostate cancer. By "blocking" that gene, malignant cells may be more vulnerable to radiation. Cancer Research UK, the British research organization, was impressed with the research done to date. Prostate cancer kills ten thousand men yearly in the Great Britain, so this is an important development.

According to the BBC, "using new technology, RNA interference, the team are able to switch off a single one of a cell's 35,000 genes. RNA uses small molecules to 'stand in the way' of specific genes to stop them working."[8]

One of the exciting prospects, according to the scientists who are working on this technique, is that it can be used after the cancer has become resistant to hormone therapy, which happens after a period of hormonal treatments. An important note: this is early, early research.

Europe and the PSA test

For some years, watchful waiting has been the prevalent "treatment" in Europe for men with slow-growing cancers (low Gleason scores). Now, some experts are suggesting that will change; that the PSA test will be used more and more to do what American doctors have done with it: to screen earlier and to treat earlier. We will have to wait and see.

Hormone therapy developments in Denmark

In September 2003, the European Cancer Conference (ECCO) met in Copenhagen, and, among many interesting reports, heard about hormone therapy being applied in a new way. This breakthrough has now been incorporated into some of the NCI's reports, so it's affecting how hormone therapy is being thought about in the United States.

Hormone therapy for Stage III or IV prostate cancer can slow the growth of cells, though in advanced cancer that has metastasized to bone or far parts of the body, very little can be done to stop the cancer, and men eventually become resistant to the hormones. That's why the gene therapy just described is useful and exciting.

But at ECCO, there is a triumphant claim that hormone therapy can actually increase survival. Or, as one article put it, "Hormone therapy combined with earlier detection is dramatically cutting the death rates from breast and prostate cancer in Europe, a British researcher said. 'The decreases in mortality parallel those seen in the United States, said Professor Richard Peto, PhD, Oxford University, United Kingdom, reporting on an analysis of a host of studies carried out over the past 40 years.'"[9]

But the difference is that, in the United States, no reputable source attributes the decline in deaths from prostate cancer to any particular therapy. And that's a big difference!

The report ("Breast and Prostate Cancer: 10-Year Survival Gains in the Hormonal Adjuvant Treatment Trials") starts by looking back at previous studies involving a total of five thousand men. As often happens in the research business, individual studies may not show much advance or retreat. In other words, they may not be conclusive. A "metastudy" looks at the other investigations as a group, and makes conclusions based on the larger number of subjects involved.

This, concludes Dr. Peto, shows that "Early hormone treatment—instead of waiting until the disease progressed—decreased the 10-year mortality risk by one-third.

"The trials were widely held to have proved that [hormone treatment] didn't save lives, but when you put them all together, they prove the opposite," he said. "Overall, hormone treatment works ridiculously well."

A word of caution: combining the results of trials done under different circumstances and under different protocols can pose a difficulty. Meta-studies sometimes come up with spurious results.

However, there are other indications that hormone therapy may be more fruitful than previously acknowledged: A British Web site—"PharmaReport" (www.leaddiscovery.co.uk/pharmareport), which looks to be a financial guide for drug companies—has a long report advising pharmaceutical companies to look to hormone therapy as a great opportunity for their corporations in the coming decade. This is mainly support for the idea that "intermittent therapy," i.e., short-term use of hormones over a long period, will improve a prostate cancer patient's quality of life by cutting down on adverse side effects.

The same article makes an ardent statement about another, more powerful kind of treatment. Once the effect of hormone therapy wears off ("hormone refractory prostate cancer"), as it is bound to do, there has been almost nothing to both reduce the size of the tumors and to prolong life.

But PharmaReport suggests that some American, British, and French studies are pointing the way to a cytotoxin called Taxotere that is "well tolerated" and "significantly reduced the risk of death by 13 percent in men with hormone refractory metastatic" prostate cancer. It also did a wonderful job in reducing pain, and was "well tolerated" by those studied.

According to the report, this is the "first time any drug has shown an extension in survival." I am happy to end this chapter with what sounds like a possible more rosy future for those afflicted with metastatic disease.

IN A SENTENCE:

> Scientists in Europe are making advances in finding powerful tools to fight prostate cancer.

Moving On

I WOULD hope that by the time you have read this book and done a lot of research and decision making, by the time you've talked to various people, you will have begun the journey toward ridding yourself of any remnant of shame or embarrassment associated in your mind with prostate cancer.

Too many men are carrying around those little malignant cells for you to feel shame.

Too many men have experienced moderate or total impotence for you to feel embarrassed about finding a pill or other treatment for yours.

Too many men have found their sex lives changed for you to be unable to discuss sex with your wife or partner—and get on track again.

But even if shame is no longer with you, it doesn't mean that you have totally moved on from this experience. In fact, you may never totally do so.

You can work on giving up the concept that you're a person with cancer, that you're "ill," that you "are" your prostate cancer. But you may have remnants for a long time of the feelings you had when you were the person experiencing diagnosis, treatment, and any repercussions of that treatment.

The person who woke up in the middle of the night and said, "My God, I'm going to die." The person who felt angry and rejected by his body when he couldn't get an erection. The person who felt that his wife was upset with him because he complained all the time, or worried all the time.

"That person" is the one who was ill.

I said, *"was."*

You are not ill now.

You had prostate cancer, but it is no longer there. It has been removed or reduced or paralyzed in some permanent or semipermanent way. You need to let go of it.

How support groups can help you—or you, them

It may be hard to recall and change back to your old, precancerous mental state now that you have been living in a state of siege. You may have forgotten what "normal" is for you. You may even have viewed cancer as such a wake-up call that you don't feel right about returning to what used to be normal for you.

If you have some leftover humiliation or discomfort about prostate cancer, if you still wake up anxious, if you're unable to fulfill your daily tasks with a mind free from doubt and anger—now that a year is almost up, you may want to seek out one of those support groups that I've talked about, you know, the ones you haven't attended yet. There, other men—in exactly the same situation as you—come together to discuss many, many issues that they have about fear, survival, readjustment, and so on.

Just as you could have used a support group before deciding on treatment, to help make decisions or cope with side effects, you can use one now—one whose membership includes men who have emerged from treatment—to help you get on with your life, to deal with all the questions that haven't yet been answered.

Maybe sharing something you've gone through and moved on from could even help someone else, at this point.

Now that's a thought! Think of the opportunities to help someone else. You could be . . . a mentor!

Becoming a mentor

Even though you might attend a group to get support for yourself, one of the things you will discover when you do go to such groups is that they are attended to some degree by novices, if you will—those who have just begun their journey through the wilds of this disease and its treatment.

Remember how it felt when you took the first steps along this journey. Having once been a questioning, somewhat scared, newly diagnosed patient yourself, you now may be able to give support to others.

And, boy, does that feel good!

It probably hasn't yet occurred to you what you have learned—and will continue learning—about prostate cancer is as valuable to others as it is for you. And that providing that information to others could be as valuable for *you* as for them. How? If you still feel some twinges of a punctured self-esteem, comforting and advising someone else who needs more help than you do will give you worlds of perspective about how far you have actually come . . . and inspiration to move forward still more.

How the world looks at you now

Earlier in this book, I talked about sharing the fact that you have cancer with colleagues or friends. I suggested that it is worthwhile to do so because talking about your illness can relieve you of some shame and depression, and because it's good to get support from people around you.

But there are exceptions to this suggestion, and I want to deal briefly with them here. How strangers or prospective employers or insurance companies see someone who has or has had prostate cancer is a different matter than how your friends may do so. Your prostate cancer and its treatment may not be hurting you at all, may not be interfering with your work—or your potential to work—but that's not necessarily how others will view you.

One of the ways to be treated as someone who is not ill, who is not less competent than before, is for you to *feel* just as competent. Your own mental attitude will definitely help mold the way others see you. It is important to do as much as you can rather than to beg off tasks, using the cancer or its treatment's side effects as an easy excuse to not disengage from your team, professionally or socially (of course, if you are truly hampered by a side effect, or need time off to go for medical appointments, that is another story). As in any work or social situation, even if cancer is not in the equation, someone who says no too often stops being asked. You need to appear vibrantly in the picture. If you don't want to be labeled a victim, don't label yourself a victim. (And telling anyone who really doesn't need to know, that you are a "cancer survivor" may do just that. People may interpret such an unsolicited announcement as designating weakness, not renewed strength.)

Also, in some circumstances, such as applying for a new job, being tactful (read, "silent") about your supposed "handicap" is not a bad idea. This is particularly true in a labor market where age is already a handicap to being hired, despite laws against such practices.

Should you apply for health or life insurance, it is likely that you will be asked if you have any diseases. It is illegal for you to answer untruthfully; and it is ill advised, since you will not get your benefits if you do so. But there is no reason for you to volunteer your prostate cancer if not asked. And there is every reason to downplay its seriousness—especially if you have Stage I or II cancer—because, as you have learned here, it may not be serious. Insurance company agents may not be up on the latest statistics about mortality. Particularly if you are only seeing your doctor for checkups, that's all they need to know about your appointments: that they are checkups.

IN A SENTENCE:

Move on: give yourself permission to no longer feel—*or* be—*ill.*

learning

Prostate Cancer on the Internet

Why turn to the Internet for information?

It has been the purpose of this book to give you as much information as I know about prostate cancer. But it must have been clear that even the most expert experts are still making very important decisions about your disease. For this reason alone, it would be worth it to continue learning about prostate cancer.

But it's also clear that your age, the stage and aggressiveness of your cancer, and the advice you receive from friends and family all play a role in what you will decide to do about screening and treatment. I cannot possibly give you all the alternatives, nor make up your mind for you. Nor do I want to.

So, continued learning is almost mandatory. And as informational tools go, the Internet is the most up-to-date resource you can consult. Even if you personally don't like to use computers, someone in your circle or family does, so get them to help you learn how to go online and to use search engines to find the data or organizations you need. If you don't own a computer, you can use those at your local public library for free. Some libraries even offer free tutorials on how to search online. You're never too old to learn how to use this invaluable resource.

Here are some tips:

Getting the most from a search engine

There are literally millions of responses when you "google" the words "prostate cancer." I just did it and got 3,370,000. (For those to whom the word "Google" is an unknown: it refers to a "search engine" on the Internet, an almost instantaneous means of finding Web sites. To reach the Google search engine, you type "www.google.com" into the horizontal "address" bar at the top of your Internet screen, and then tap "Go" onscreen or the "Enter" key on your keyboard. Another popular search engine is the one at "www.yahoo.com.")

When you use a search engine, you have to choose your search words carefully. For instance, when I typed the phrases (and always put phrases in quotes) "prostate cancer" and "chat rooms" into the Search bar, I got the following response:

> "Results 1–10 of about 24,400 for 'prostate cancer' 'chat rooms'. (0.41 seconds)"

Listed below this box were "links" to the first—and most popular—ten Web sites that contained both the phrases. (Tapping your cursor on a link brings you directly to the Web page described. To return to the search engine listings, tap your cursor on "Back" at the top of the Internet screen.) The first sites that are listed may not be quite what you were looking for . . . but you have another 23,390 to go! The chances are, if you choose your search terms well, you won't have to scan through more than a dozen or two responses to find useful information, so don't be daunted by the total number of results.

The more phrases or words, or more specific the terms, you type into the search engine, the more specific your responses will be. In fact, if you put enough words in, you may get back a response that says, "There are no pages with all these words" or something like that.

That is why the scattergun approach may not always be the best one for finding Web sites that will answer your questions.

A more directed approach

I found it more useful to start by imagining what organizations or institutions in the medical world might be helpful to me in learning about a topic. Thus, the National Institutes of Health come to mind. Or the National Cancer Institute. Or the American Cancer Society. Or Centers for Disease Control. By typing those phrases into the search engine (one at a time), I soon came to the official Web sites of the NIH or the NCI or the ACS or the CDC (see Resources).

Each of those sites has its own search engine, which allows you to find "prostate cancer" references on that site alone. Pretty soon, you will have narrowed your search to those organizations' specific pages about your special realm of inquiry.

What institutional sites omit

What you don't get from this kind of search are the rumors, myths, far-out ideas, and unofficial news and information on prostate cancer. Even though the NCI and ACS now talk about CAM, for instance, some years back they might not have done so. To get to that kind of information, you may need to start back at Google (or Yahoo!, or other search engines . . .) and string together not lucid phrases but combinations of terms—called keywords—that are as pinpointed as you can make them, such as Complementary Medicine Prostate Cancer Europe. This technique brings up all Internet documents containing those words, ranked by those most popularly requested.

If you are unaccustomed to thinking up keywords, it may be helpful to you to see some of the answers that come up when you do this kind of thing, so that you don't use too general a term that brings forth a lot of articles having nothing whatsoever to do with your search. Be aware that words used in slightly different forms, such as singular versus plural, may bring up different articles, as the search engine is absolutely literal about the commands. So, for instance, typing "PSA test" and "PSA testing" may yield different results. Keep in mind, too, that individual words such as "prostate" and "cancer" can show up widely separated in an article or research paper, so that if you want individual words to always show up as whole phrases, always put quotation marks around the entire phrase. This way, the search engine will bring you only those pages or sites that have the phrase exactly as you have it between marks.

You can also type in a distinctive phrase from a quote that you have read somewhere, such as in a newspaper (again, place it between quotation marks), and the search engine will quickly give you the exact location(s) where that quote can be found. That way, you'll be able to verify the source of some statements you've read out of context or without credits for the writer/speaker.

If you're looking for what are called "chat rooms" on the Internet—a chance to trade questions, answers, and comments with anonymous patients who have the same disease as you—that can be accomplished through a search engine, too. Some sites may not have real-time chat rooms but do offer a bulletin board where you may post questions and also read what others have posted. You may now be knowledgeable about prostate cancer to the point that you may even be able to answer someone else's posted query!

How Internet search results look onscreen

Here are some examples of what my searches turned up, pretty much in the form in which I read them (the listing may have changed a little since), so that you can see what typical search engine results will look like. Search engines pick up only a small amount of descriptive text, thus the ellipses ending some entries.

www.nutrition2000.com
Cancer Message Boards Share stories, advice & fears with other young adults here.

www.PlanetCancer.org
Prostate-Help Patients Helping Patients . . . Chat Rooms: This is the same as before with no changes and is where we hold our . . . grouping of things that will allow one to search about prostate cancer

www.prostate-help.net/
Shared Experience Cancer Support—Cancer Chat Rooms and Newsgroup . . .

Some other examples of chat Rooms

The following chat rooms are for prostate cancer and can all be subscribed to.

www.sharedexperience.org/chatrooms.lasso
Prostate Cancer Overview . . . Links to mailing lists, Usenet, and chat rooms. News: There are many prostate-cancer news sites and e-mail and regular-mail newsletters (some of which are free). . . .

www.hypertext.org/ENGLISH/OVER.html
Prostate Cancer E-Community—Chat Rooms
A gateway to the Prostate Cancer online community. Share Prostate Cancer experiences. Chat Rooms. . . .

www.pccnc.org/ecommunity/chat_rooms.shtml
Chat rooms can be either "live" chats or bulletin board-type chats . . . to discuss clinical and nonclinical issues about prostatitis, BPH, and prostate cancer. . . .

www.onconurse.com/factsheets/prostate_resources.html
Chat Rooms—Trustworthy, Physician-Reviewed Information from . . . Learn more, Chat Rooms. Want to talk to other members in real time? . . . Parkinson's. Pregnancy (5). Prostate Cancer. Relationships Support. Self Injury. Sexual Conditions . . .

content.health.msn.com/community/chat_rooms/default.htm
HealingWell.com Community . . . 12:46 PM. Chat Rooms Open, Admin, 2, 251, Admin 9/8/2004 9:25 AM. Prostate Cancer Resources, Admin, 2, 386, Admin 4/2/2004 1:40 PM. PC or Prostatis . . .

www.healingwell.com/community/default.aspx F=35
HealingWell.com—Resource Directory: Prostate_Cancer Prostate Cancer Resource Center . . . articles, patient stories, community message boards and chat rooms, books, free . . .

www.healingwell.com/pages/Prostate_Cancer/
The Cancer Survivors Network, supplying information, resources
. . . Chat Rooms: To access the chat room, you must register on
CSN and log in. Having trouble entering a CSN Chat Room? . . .
Pituitary Cancer, 5, Prostate Cancer, 1358, . . .

www.acscsn.org/Forum/Discussion/summary.html

Looking for clinical trials?

This can be accomplished, too. A Web page from the American Cancer
Society allows you to put in your particular profile and actually find a clinical trial—if there is one—that fits your needs (go to www.clinicaltrials
.cancer.org).

.Org vs. .com

As I mentioned way back in this book, it is worth keeping in mind that
an Internet address that ends .org (as in cancer.org) is a nonprofit organization. One that ends .com (as in "commercial," or for profit) is not. That
doesn't mean that all nonprofits tell it like it is, and no .coms do, but you're
much more likely to get better medical information from an .org. PS: If you
run into an "edu," that means it's an educational organization, such as a
university-run Web site—and that's good. And .gov means it's a government
site . . . not so good for CAM studies, but good for conventional information.

The Dartmouth Atlas

Don't forget my earlier reference to the value of the Dartmouth Atlas.
Type the following into the address box on your computer's browser:
www.dartmouthatlas.org.
When the site comes up, go to Search on the home page.
Type in "prostate cancer" and you'll get a lot of information on what kind
of treatments are being done in which localities.

Other Web sites to check out

In the Resource section that follows this chapter, there are a lot of Web addresses that can be useful. Here are some that I found particularly helpful:

○ The National Cancer Institute: www.cancer.gov
○ A dictionary of cancer terms: www.cancer.gov/dictionary
○ A page where you can get actual "live" information from cancer specialists. Look for "LiveHelp" on the NCI's site.
○ A site aimed specifically at older people with eyesight problems or limited acquaintance with the Internet: http://nihseniorhealth.gov/prostatecancer/toc.html
○ A site about impotence: www.impotence-guide.com/impotence-causes.html

And these kinds of links—of which there are hundreds—at the Web sites of the organizations I've placed in parentheses:

○ Brief Hormone Therapy Boosts Prostate Cancer Survival (American Cancer Society)
○ Exercise May Help Men Beat Fatigue from Prostate Radiation (American Cancer Society)
○ FDA Approves New Indication for Taxotere—Prostate Cancer (Food and Drug Administration)
○ First Evidence That Chemotherapy Extends Life in Advanced Prostate Cancer (National Cancer Institute)
○ First Prostate Cancer Prevention Drug Found, but Not All Men Benefit (National Cancer Institute)
○ Prostate Cancer Outcomes Study (National Cancer Institute)
○ Rapid Rise in PSA May Predict Aggressive Prostate Cancer (American Cancer Society)
○ Some Men with Low PSAs Have Prostate Cancer (National Cancer Institute) Vasectomy and Cancer Risk (National Cancer Institute)

One final note about Web searches. You'll often get an "address" that has the following as a "prefix:" http://www or just the www. You seldom need the http://, and often you can enter the address without the "www," too. But do take care typing the body of the rest of the address, as the slightest difference in spelling, wording, or punctuation may bring up a totally different site than the one you are requesting. If you want to return to a site with a long address, or want to remember where you read something, print out the first page of its home page. The printout will include the complete address of the site, for you to refer to later.

IN A SENTENCE:

> *The Internet is a terrific tool for locating prostate cancer–related resources.*

Glossary

ACUPUNCTURE: The insertion of long needles at various points in the body to interfere with the conveyance of pain along the nerves. Originating in China, and centuries old, this has become a fairly common "alternative" practice in the United States, along with chiropractic and massage.

ALLOPATHIC MEDICINE: A term synonymous with "standard western medicine," i.e., the kind of practice of medicine that has been used in Western nations for several hundred years.

ALTERNATIVE MEDICINE: See "Complementary medicine."

ANALGESIC: A painkiller.

ANDROGENS: Any compound that affects masculine behavior and characteristics is an androgen. Testosterone is an androgen, but there are others.

ANECDOTAL EVIDENCE: Stories and hearsay about the positive effects of food or medicine or treatment that is not backed up by rigorous studies.

ANTIOXIDANT: "Antioxidants" are any substance that helps retard or stop oxidation in the body. These are present in many vegetables with yellow colors, and have shown some ability to retard the growth of cancerous cells.

AROMATHERAPY: The use of odors to help heal the mind and the body.

BENIGN: Not cancerous.

BIOFEEDBACK: In general, the practice of paying attention to the feelings or actions of the body (such as blood pressure, heartbeat, heat and cold) so as to control those functions with the mind.

BIOPSY: A procedure in which a hollow needle is inserted into a part of the body to pull out a tiny sample which is then sent to a pathologist for examination.

CAM: See "complementary medicine."

CARCINOGENS: Known environmental causes of any particular kind of cancer, such as smoking or PCBs.

CHRONIC: A chronic condition or disease is one that will be with you for the rest of your life but will most likely simply need to be watched and periodically treated, as opposed to a "terminal" disease. Diabetes, multiple sclerosis, and athlete's foot (to name but a few, in a range of seriousness) are chronic conditions.

COMPLEMENTARY MEDICINE: The current term for the use of medications or practices other than standard "Western" treatments. Sometimes called Complementary and Alternative Medicine (CAM) or, simply, Alternative Medicine.

CONTRAST MATERIAL: Any of a number of liquid compounds used to make parts of your body show lighter in X-rays or CAT scans. Some of this is imbibed (flavored with mint or orange) and some is injected into your veins.

CONVENTIONAL MEDICINE: Medical practices as practiced trained and licensed MDs, Dos, physical therapists, psychologists, and registered nurses.

CT SCAN: Computerized Tomography, commonly called CAT scan. A sophisticated type of X-ray device that captures images of "slices" of the body in a few minutes.

DIGITAL RECTAL EXAM (DRE): A procedure in which the doctor inserts a gloved finger into the rectum to examine the rectum and prostate to look for an irregular or abnormally firm area, helps to gauge tumor size, and it may show if the cancer has spread into nearby tissues.

DILATION: Opening up of a vessel or connective tube.

DNA: The material that controls genetic transmission.

DOUBLE-BLIND STUDY: The so-called "gold standard" of protocols, this is when two or more groups of patients are used, each one getting a different drug or treatment, and neither group knowing which is the experimental or trial one. Results are compared by researchers.

ENDEMIC: Built-in, part of the organism, born with.

ENDOSCOPE: One of several varieties of tubes that are inserted into either the throat or rectum to see what's going on inside. The most sophisticated is a long, flexible fiber-optic tube, used to examine the colon in a colonoscopy.

ENZYME: A complex protein that acts to help complete biochemical changes in the body.

EPIDIDYMIS: A long, coiled tube that stores and matures the semen from the testes.

ERECTILE DYSFUNCTION: See "Impotence."

ESTROGEN: Hormone that determines feminine characteristics.

EXTERNAL-BEAM RADIATION: The use of powerful X-rays to destroy cells within the body.

FALSE POSITIVE, FALSE NEGATIVE: Tests that deliver results that later turn out to be inaccurate.

IMPOTENCE: The inability to get a partial or full erection. Also called "erectile dysfunction."

INCONTINENCE: Usually defined as the inability to keep from urinating. Sometimes also used for other lack of sphincter control, as in "bowel incontinence."

INFORMED CONSENT: You have the right to understand your treatment and to say whether you want it or not.

IODIZED: Anything that is treated with iodine.

LAPRYSCOPICALLY: A lapryscopic operation is one done through several tiny incisions with miniaturized instruments, so as to minimize the trauma caused by large incisions.

MALIGNANT: Cancerous, cells that are growing abnormally.

MARKER: An indication that one of your genes has the capacity to create a disease.

METASTASES: Cancer that has spread from one part of the body—its seat of origin—into other parts. "Metastasizing" is the verb form.

METASTASIZING: When cancer spreads from its original seat of origin into other parts of the body.

MODALITIES: A synonym for "types" of treatment.

MUTATION: Any change in the DNA of a cell. Mutations may be caused by mistakes during cell division, or they may be caused by exposure to DNA-damaging agents in the environment. Mutations can be harmful, beneficial, or have no effect. Certain mutations may lead to cancer or other diseases.

ONCOLOGIST: A physician who specializes in cancer.

PALLIATIVE: Any treatment or therapies that are designed primarily to relieve pain and other uncomfortable symptoms of a disease rather than to slow down or stop the disease.

PARASYMPATHETIC: That part of the nervous system that slows down heartbeats, dilates blood vessels and otherwise slows down physiological functions. As contrasted with the "sympathetic nervous system."

PATHOLOGIST: A doctor who studies and identifies the cell and tissue changes produced by disease.

PLACEBO: A fake pill or other treatment that is given to one group of patients in a double-blind study to compare with the real treatment that is given to a different group of patients.

POLYPHENOLS: Polyphenols are chemicals found in some plants or vegetables that have an "antioxidant" capability.

PROGNOSIS: A prediction as to the course and extent of an illness.

PROPRIETARY: Refers to drugs or equipment that is the property of a corporation or profit-making institution.

PROSTATE-SPECIFIC ANTIGEN: A protein generated within the prostate gland normally. Its leakage in large quantities into the bloodstream may be an indication that a man has prostate cancer.

PROSTATIC HYPERPLASIA: When your prostate increases in size.

PROSTATITIS: When the prostate becomes inflamed. Often the result of viral or bacterial infection, prostatitis can make a man need to urinate often, and can cause pain in the genitourinary organs or groin.

PROSTHETIC: Any imitation or synthetic device used to simulate a body part, for practical, psychological, or aesthetic considerations. For instance: a prosthetic breast, a prosthetic leg, a prosthetic eye.

PROTEIN: One of several kinds of molecules that are essential for certain bodily functions.

PSYCHOPHARMACOLOGIST: A psychiatrist who specializes in choosing the proper medication for psychological or psychiatric problems—ranging from outright psychosis to sleep problems to anxiety and depression.

QUALITY OF LIFE: This term has taken on a special meaning in recent years. It refers to the fact that some people, faced with a chronic or terminal illness, are as interested in how their emotional health is maintained as they are in cure; in their ability to communicate with loved ones; in their spiritual well-being.

RADIUM: A radioactive element.

RANDOMIZED: The practice in a double-blind study of using two groups of patients, randomly assigned, one group receiving treatment of one kind; the other receiving a different kind of treatment.

REMISSION: A period of time in which symptoms and pathologic indications of your cancer have disappeared. As contrasted with "cure," remission usually means that physicians cannot say whether the cancer will return or not.

RETROSPECTIVE STUDY: A review of literature dating back several years, and collected from various sources. Often called a "metastudy."

SEMINAL VESICLES: Tubes containing a fluid that nourishes sperm; the sperm is stored here after leaving the epididymis.

SPHINCTER: Muscles that close openings in the anus and the urethra, allowing evacuation to be under your control.

STAGING: Term used for determining how far your cancer has advanced in your body.

SUPPORT GROUP: Any of a variety of assemblies of people who have had a similar disease, who get together to share feelings and problems.

SYMPATHETIC: That part of the nervous system that speeds up the heart, constricts blood vessels, and so forth; part of the "flight or fright" system in the human being.

TENS: Stands for transcutaneous electrical nerve stimulation. A battery-powered device, the small pointed wand delivers low electrical impulses that act like acupuncture needles to interfere with the transmission of pain.

TERMINAL: This refers to diseases that will most likely kill you, or which are in the final phase.

TESTICLES: Official name: testes. Sperm is produced in these oval-shaped glands. So is testosterone.

TESTOSTERONE: The male hormone that is responsible for many male physical characteristics; also suspected of being responsible for some male behavior characteristics as well, especially violence.

TRUS: Transrectal Urethral Screening. The use of ultrasound as a diagnostic tool for prostate cancer.

TURP: Surgery that makes the opening through which urine runs, larger. Needed for BPH, which creates "bladder outlet obstruction."

URETHRA: A passage way from your bladder to the end of your penis. It also carries sperm and seminal fluid when you ejaculate.

VAS DEFERENS: A channel that takes sperm from the epididymis to the seminal vesicles.

VASECTOMY: Cutting the vase deferens for the purpose of sterilization.

YOGA: A practice, centuries old, that establishes both physical and mental calm through exercises and meditation.

Notes

Introduction and Day 1

1. Figures such as these—found throughout this book—are taken from a variety of government organizations. In this case, it's the National Cancer Institute. The specific study for these figures—SEER (Surveillance, Epidemiology, and End Results)—has been researching prostate cancer for some time.

Day 2

1. The paperback came out in 1970, published by Simon & Schuster.
2. The National Cancer Institute (NCI) web site (www.cancer.com) has a huge amount of material. This figure came from that web site.

Day 3

1. NCI Web site.
2. National Prostate Cancer Coalition.

Day 5

1. www.saltlakeregional.com/second/urological/options.htm.
2. American Cancer Society is one of several important national non-profit organizations focusing on cancer. They issue book-

lets, do public service spots, and have an 800 number (1-800-ACS 2345) and a Web site: www.cancer.org.
3. James Strickler, Dartmouth Medical Center.
4. http://health.yahoo.com/search/healthnews?lb=s&p=id%3A65334.
5. *Fortune Magazine,* November 2004.

Day 6

1. NCI web site.
2. NCI web site.
3. US TOO, a support group for patients with prostate cancer and their families (www.ustoo.com).4. NCI.

Day 7

1. NCI Web site.

Week 2

1. NCI web site.
2. NCI Web site.
3. Hanyu Ni, PhD, MPH; Catherine Simile, PhD; Ann M. Hardy, DrPH "Utilization of Complementary and Alternative Medicine by United States Adults: Results from the 1999 National Health Interview Survey," *Medical Care* 40, no. 4 (April 2002): 353–8.
4. Medcomres.com.
5. Mary Ann Richardson, Tina Sanders, J. Lynn Palmer, Anthony Greisinger, S. Eva Singletary, "Complementary/Alternative Medicine Use in a Comprehensive Cancer Center and the Implications for Oncology," *Journal of Clinical Oncology* 20, no. 13 (July 1, 2002) 2505–2514.
6. NCI Web site.
7. NCI Web site.

Week 3

1. NCI Web site.
2. L. A. G. Ries, M. P. Eisner, C. L. Kosary, et al., eds., *SEER Cancer Statistics Review, 1975–2001*, National Cancer Institute. Bethesda, MD, http://seer.cancer.gov/csr/1975_2001/, 2004.

Week 4

1. *The New York Times*, Dec. 14, 2004.

Month 2

1. *Cancer* 101, n0.3: 550–7.
2. American Cancer Society.

3. American Cancer Society.
4. This and other valuable information about health and medicine can be found in *The Merck Manual of Diagnosis and Therapy*, Rahway, NJ: Merck Publishing, 2000). 5. For more, see the NCI site.
6. The American Heart Association web site says, "Omega-3 fatty acids benefit the heart of healthy people, and those at high risk of—or who have—cardiovascular disease. **We recommend eating fish (particularly fatty fish) at least two times a week.** Fish is a good source of protein and doesn't have the high saturated fat that fatty meat products do. Fatty fish like mackerel, lake trout, herring, sardines, albacore tuna and salmon are high in two kinds of omega-3 fatty acids, **eicosapentaenoic acid (EPA)** and **docosahexaenoic acid (DHA)."**
7. http://archives.foodsafetynetwork.ca/ffnet/2003/8–2003/functional_food-net_august_11.htm.
8. NCI Web site.

Month 3

1. www.psa-rising.com/med/prevention/lycopene_PIN04.html.
2. www.psa-rising.com/med/prevention/lycopene_PIN04.html.

Month 4

1. www.nci.nih.gov/cancertopics/understanding-prostate-cancer-treatment/page 5.

Month 5

1. ." Christopher Lukas and Henry M. Seiden, Ph.D, *Silent Grief: Living in the Wake of Suicide* (New Jersey: Jason Aronson, 1997).
2. www.selfhelpweb.org.
3. AllRefer—a dot-com on the internet that deals with a wide variety of health issues.
4. Karen Kaplan, MPH, Sc.D. and Christopher Lukas, *Staying In Charge: Practical Plans for the End of Your Life* (New York: John Wiley and Sons, 2004).

Month 6

1. Linda Emanuel, MD, personal communication.

Month 7

1. http://en.mimi.hu/sexuality/sex_drive.html.
2. webhealthcentre.com.
3. *Charette A. Dersch, Steven M. Harris, Thomas Kimball, et al., "Sexual Issues for Aging Adults," Texas Tech University* (www.hs.ttu.edu/sexuality&aging/).

4. *ibid.*
5. There are innumerable references to oxytocin in the popular media these days. This particular quote came from http://www.exceptionalmarriage.com/new_page_5.htm
6. *Merck Manual.*

Month 8

1. NCI Web site.
2. Ian M. Thompson, M.D., Phyllis J. Goodman, M.S., Catherine M. Tangen, Dr.P.H., et al. "The Influence of Finasteride on the Development of Prostate Cancer," *New England Journal of Medicine*, June 4, 2003.
3. NCI Web site
4. NCI Web site
5. NCI Web site
6. www.cancer.med.umich.edu/prostcan/spore.htm.
7. NCI Web site

Month 9

1. NCI Web site
2. The Cancer Information Network, "a noncommercial site founded to provide support and information to cancer patients and their caregivers. It is our desire to provide patients with the latest high-quality information from reputable sources and the tools to decipher and organize that information. The Network is founded on the belief that proactive patients who educate themselves to take an active role in decisions regarding their therapy can effect their outcome in a positive way."

Month 10

1. The December 2004 issue.

Month 11

1. http://menshealth.about.com/od/prostatehealth/.
2. www.4men.org.
3. www.edap-hifu.com/eng/physicians/hifu/3a_treatment_overview.htm.
4. news.bbc.co.uk/2/hi/health/3944269.stm.
5. www.docguide.com/.

For Further Reading

Alterowitz, Ralph and Barbara. *Intimacy with Impotence: The Couple's Guide to Better Sex after Prostate Disease*. New York, Perseus Books Group, 2004.

Alterowitz, Ralph and Barbara. *The Lovin' Ain't Over: The Couple's Guide to Better Sex After Prostate Disease*. New York, Da Capo Press, 2004.

Arnot, Dr. Bob. *The Prostate Cancer Protection Plan: The Foods, Supplements, and Drugs that Can Combat Prostate Cancer*. Boston. Little, Brown, 2001.

Bennet M, Lengacher C. "Use of Complementary Therapies in a Rural Cancer Population." *Oncology Nursing Forum* 1999; 26(8):1287, 1294.

Bostwick, David G. (Ed.) *American Cancer Society's Complete Guide to Prostate Cancer*. Washington, D.C., American Cancer Society.

Cassileth, B. and C. Chapman. "Alternative and Complementary Cancer Therapies," *Cancer* 1996; 77(6):1026.

Clark, Nancy, MS, RD. *Sports and Nutrition Guidebook*, 2nd edition. Champaign, IL, Human Kinetics Publishers. 2003.

Eisenberg D. M., R. B. Davis, S. L. Ettner, et al. "Trends in Alternative medicine use in the United States." *Journal of the American Medical Association*. 1990.

Grimm, Peter, John Blasko, and John Sylvester. *The Prostate Cancer Treatment Book*. New York. McGraw-Hill, 2003.

Kantoff, Philip, ed. *Prostate Cancer: Principles and Practice*. Lippincott Williams & Wilkins, 2002.

Kao, G. D. and P. Devine. "Use of Complementary Health Practices by Prostate Carcinoma Patients Undergoing Radiation Therapy." *Cancer* 2000; 88(3):615.

Kaplan, Karen MPH, ScD, and Christopher Lukas. *Staying in Charge.* New York. John Wiley & Sons. 2004.

Klein, Eric A., ed., and Ralph A. Straffon. *Management of Prostate Cancer,* 2nd edition. Totowa, NJ. Humana Press. 2003.

Laken, Virginia and Keith. *Making Love Again: Hope for Couples Facing Loss of Sexual Intimacy.* Westport, CT. Dialogue Press, 2002

Lange, Paul H. and Christine Adamec. *Prostate Cancer for Dummies.* New York. For Dummies, 2002.

Marks, Sheldon, MD. *Prostate and Cancer: A Family Guide to Diagnosis, Treatment and Survival,* 3rd edition. Perseus Publishing, 2003.

Nelson, W. "Alternative Cancer Treatments," *Oncology Practice* 1998; 15(4):85–93.

Nixon, Daniel and Max Gomez. *The Prostate Health Program: A Guide to Preventing and Controlling Prostate Cancer.* Free Press, 2004.

Oesterling, Joseph A. and Mark A. Moyad. *The ABC's of Prostate Cancer: The Book That Could Save Your Life.* New York. J.W. Ann Arbor. J. W. Edwards, Inc. 1997.

Richardson, M. A. and S. E. Straus. "Complementary and Alternative Medicine: Opportunities and Challenges for Cancer Management and Research," *Seminars in Oncology* 2002, 29(6): 531.

Richardson, M. A., T. Sanders, J. L. Palmer, et al. *Prostate Diet Cookbook.* Harbor Press, 2001.

Simile, C., and A. M. Hardy. "Utilization of Complementary and Alternative Medicine By United States Adults: Results from the 1999 National Health Interview Survey." *Medical Care* 2002; 40(4):353

Sparber, A., L. Bauer, G. Curt, et al. "Use of Complementary Medicine by Adult Patients Participating in Cancer Clinical Trials," *Oncology Nursing Forum* 2000; 27(4):623.

Strum, Stephen B. and Donna Pogliano. *A Primer on Prostate Cancer: The Empowered Patient's Guide,* October 1, 2002.

Sugarman, Sally Sower. *Choices: Living with Cancer, Dying with Dignity.* Free booklet download as .pdf from http://psa-rising.com/books/choices.htm

Walsh, Patrick, MD and Janet Farrar Worthington. *Dr. Patrick Walsh's Guide to Surviving Prostate Cancer.* New York. Warner Books, 2002.

White, J. D. "Complementary, Alternative, and Unproven Methods of Cancer Treatment." In *Cancer: Principles and Practice of Oncology,* 6th edition, DeVita, Hellman, Rosenberg, eds. Philadelphia: Lippincott Williams & Wilkins, 2001, 3147.

"Complementary and Alternative Medicine Use in a Comprehensive Cancer Center and the Implications for Oncology," *Journal of Clinical Oncology* 2000; 8(13):2505.

Other Resources

ON THE Internet and in the phone book are almost endless sources for information about cancer in general, and prostate cancer specifically. I've culled some of those that seem both useful and borderline. I advise browsing what looks interesting; it's important for you to make your own decisions about what works for you.

American Dietetic Association:
www.eatright.org

American Heart Association's Delicious Decisions:
www.deliciousdecisions.org

American Medical Association:
www.ama-assn.org

Alliance for Prostate Cancer Prevention (APCaP):
www.apcap.org
APCaP has been created to sup-port efforts to prevent the serious consequences of the disease itself for men who have not been diagnosed and are unaware of the deadly effects of prostate cancer. "The mission of APCaP is to bring public and private business leaders, legislators, health providers and administrators, researchers, federal, state and local health officials into a coordinated cohesive forum to enhance and promote prostate cancer awareness, education, research and primary and secondary prevention programs. The goal of this diversified stakeholder group is to implement and evaluate ambitious plans that are designed to eliminate prostate cancer as a health threat in the United States by 2010.

Blackhealthnet:
www.blackhealthnet.com

Calorie Control Council:
www.caloriescount.org

Cancercare.org:
1–800 4 CANCER

Cancer Information Service:
Toll-free 1–800–4–CANCER
(1–800–422–6237)
TTY (for deaf and hard of hearing callers)
1–800–332–8615

CancerSource.com:
www.cancercource.com

Centers for Disease Control:
www.cdc.gov

Consumer Nutrition Hotline:
1–800 366–1655

Consumer's Union:
www.consumersunion.org/health/
hmo-review

Food and Nutrition Information Center at the U.S. Department of Agriculture:
www.nal.usda.gov/fnic

HealthFinder:
www.healthfinder.gov

"Man to Man" Prostate Cancer Patient Education and Support
c/o American Cancer Society:
  1–800-ACS-2345, or www.cancer.org

MedLine (a service of NIH and U.S. National Library of Medicine) Publications include:
"Are You Considering Using Complementary and Alternative Medicine (CAM)?"
(http://nccam.nih.gov/health/decisions)
"Selecting a Complementary and Alternative Medicine Practitioner"
(http://nccam.nih.gov/health/practitioner)
"Consumer Financial Issues in Complementary and Alternative Medicine"
(http://nccam.nih.gov/health/)
NCCAM Clearinghouse
Post Office Box 7923

Gaithersburg, MD 20898–7923
Toll-free in the United States:
1–888–644–6226
from outside the U.S.: 301–519–3153
TTY: 1–866–464–3615
fax: 1–866–464–3616
e-mail: info@nccam.nih.gov
Web site: http://nccam.nih.gov

The Food and Drug Administration (FDA):
5600 Fishers Lane
Rockville, MD 20857
1–888–463–6332 (toll-free)
Web site: http://www.fda.gov/
The FDA regulates drugs and medical devices to ensure that they are safe and effective. This agency provides a number of publications for consumers, including information about dietary supplements.
FDA's Dietary Supplements:
Web page: http://www.cfsan.fda.gov/
~dms/supplmnt.html

The Federal Trade Commission (FTC):
Consumer Response Center
Federal Trade Commission
CRC-240 Washington, DC 20580
telephone (toll-free): 1–877-FTC-HELP
(1–877–382–4357)
TTY: 202–326–2502
Web site: http://www.ftc.gov
The FTC enforces consumer protection laws and offers publications to guide consumers, and also collects information about fraudulent claims.

National Cancer Institute Complementary and Alternative Medicine Section:
www.cancer.gov

NCI's PDQ:
A database, has information about the use of CAM in the treatment of cancer:
http://www.cancer.gov/cancerinfo/pdq/cam

For clinical trials of all sorts, go to:

www.cancer.gov/clinicaltrials

http://nccam.nih.gov/clinicaltrials/

http://www.cancer.gov/occam/trials.html

National Prostate Cancer Coalition (NPCC):
www.npcc.org
"Sets the standard for rapidly reducing the burden of prostate cancer on American men and their families through awareness, outreach, and advocacy. Its signature initiative, the Drive Against Prostate Cancer, is the only national mobile screening vehicle and aims to screen 10,000 men for free in 2004."

National Institutes of Health:
www.health.nih.gov

Nutrition Data.com:
www.nutritiondata.com

Prostate Cancer Support Group Network
c/o American Foundation for Urologic Disease
300 W. Pratt Street, Suite 401
Baltimore, MD 21201
1–800–242–2383
Web site: www.selfhelpweb.org

PSA-Rising:
www.psa-rising.com

www.Rxlaughter.com

U.S. Department of Agriculture's Center for Nutrition Policy and Promotion
www.usda.gov/cnpp

"Us Too! International, Inc." (Cancer Support Groups):
www.ustoo.org
5003 Fairview Avenue Downers Grove, IL 60515
toll-free 1–800–80-US-TOO
(1–800–808–7866)
or non-toll-free 1–630–795–1002
fax: 630–795–1602

Vegetarian Resource Group:
www.vrg.org

Weight Control Information Network:
www.niddk.nih.gov

Acknowledgments

WITHOUT THE help of my agent, Jennifer Unter, this book would never have come about.

My wife, Susan Lukas, gave me the space and time to write. To all the editors and originators of the First Year series at Marlowe & Company, but especially Suzanne McCloskey, thanks for the idea, the format, and the freedom to write as I chose.

And to all those who shared their stories with me—rest assured they are helpful to the rest of us.

Index